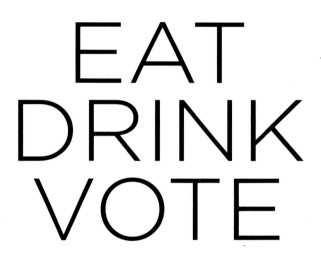

EAT
DRINK
VOTE

MARION NESTLE

BESTSELLING AUTHOR OF *WHAT TO EAT*

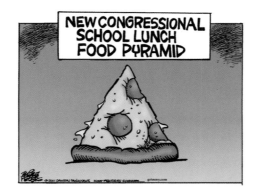

AN ILLUSTRATED GUIDE TO FOOD POLITICS

EAT
DRINK
VOTE

WITH SELECTIONS FROM THE VAULTS OF THE CARTOONIST GROUP

RODALE.

Rodale books may be purchased for business or promotional use or for special sales. For information, please write to: Special Markets Department, Rodale Inc., 733 Third Avenue, New York, NY 10017.

Printed in China

Rodale Inc. makes every effort to use acid-free ∞, recycled paper ♺.

Book design by Amy C. King and Mike Smith

Cartoon Credits: See page 192

Library of Congress Cataloging-in-Publication Data is on file with the publisher.

ISBN-13: 978-1-60961-586-4 paperback

Distributed to the trade by Macmillan

2 4 6 8 10 9 7 5 3 1 paperback

 RODALE.

We inspire and enable people to imrove their lives and the world around them.
www.rodalebooks.com

To Mal

CONTENTS

EAT DRINK VOTE

Introduction

IN 2012, THE US DEPARTMENT OF AGRICULTURE (USDA) proposed new nutrition standards for meals served in school lunch programs. These specified the numbers and sizes of food servings necessary to meet children's nutritional needs and promote health, but prevent obesity. One provision mentioned that tomato paste must meet the same volume requirements as other fruits and vegetables—one-half cup—in order to be counted as a full serving. The makers of pizza for school lunches objected. This much tomato paste would make pizza soggy, they said. How best to make the USDA reverse this decision? Go to Congress, of course. Lobbyists for school pizza makers went to work. Bingo! The Senate inserted an amendment to the agriculture spending act, which authorizes funding for all USDA programs: "None of the funds made available by this Act may be used to ... require crediting of tomato paste and puree based on volume."

The result? A dab of tomato paste on pizza now counts as a vegetable in school lunches. Kids get fewer servings of real vegetables in those lunches. Food companies now know that Congress will take care of them if they don't like federal regulations. And the public now knows that no regulation—no matter how strongly recommended by nutrition and health experts and supported by research—is too small to be overturned by Congress to please corporate constituents.

I have written about such issues in professional articles and in my books devoted to food politics, food safety, supermarket choices, pet foods, and calories. I also write about such things on my (almost) daily blog, www.foodpolitics.com and in occasional tweets @marionnestle. But political cartoonists can tell the whole story in one drawing. ▼

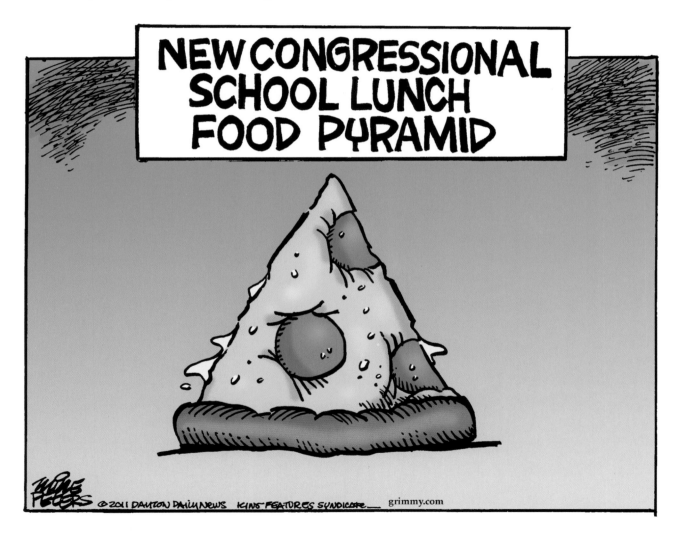

WHY AN ILLUSTRATED GUIDE TO FOOD POLITICS?

I LOVE FOOD CARTOONS. I started using them in my books in 2002 when I convinced the University of California Press to let me include a few drawings in the first edition of *Food Politics: How the Food Industry Influences Nutrition and Health*. The Press also agreed to publish cartoons in my subsequent book, *Safe Food: The Politics of Food Safety,* and in a later book on the safety of pet foods, *Pet Food Politics.* For decades, I have collected cartoons to use in my lectures to students and to the public. I am always looking for drawings that make it easier to explain complex concepts or points of view about food issues. That is how I first came across the work of some of the cartoonists represented in this book.

In 2005, for example, the USDA replaced its old pyramid-shaped guide to healthy eating, which dated to the early 1990s. The new pyramid displayed rainbow stripes but no visible food. To understand what it meant, you had to know that each stripe was supposed to represent a distinct food group. I thought the earlier pyramid (reproduced on page 53) was more effective in conveying the idea that it's better for health to eat some foods than others. Surely politics was responsible for eliminating any trace of that concept, but explaining how food lobbies exert influence over federal dietary advice can put audiences to sleep. In contrast, cartoons wake everyone up. I managed to find several cartoons dealing with the new pyramid, but this one best captured the absurdity of the new design. I still use it in talks. Whenever I show it, audiences get the point, laugh, and pay attention to the rest of my lecture. A great cartoon makes my work easier—and a lot more fun. ▶

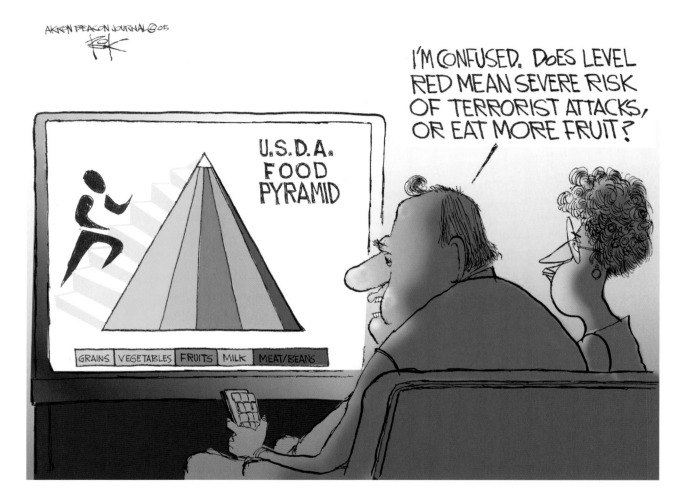

One more example: My most recent book (coauthored with Dr. Malden Nesheim) is *Why Calories Count: From Science to Politics*. It is about the most intangible of subjects. Calories cannot be seen, tasted, or smelled, and are difficult to measure accurately either in food or in the body. Mal and I struggled hard to make abstract scientific concepts accessible to general readers, and we wanted to include cartoons to lighten things up a bit. We found two that worked well. Both turned out to be drawn by Steve Kelley, who seems to have a particular interest in the same kinds of food issues that I do. ▼ ▶

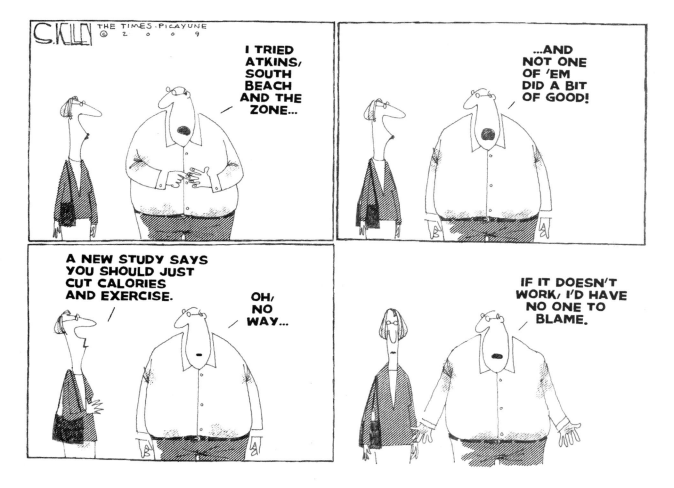

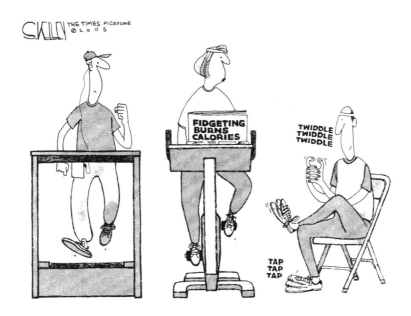

To republish Kelley's cartoons in our book, we had to obtain reprint rights to his work. This led me to the Cartoonist Group, which works with Creators Syndicate to license Kelley's drawings. The Cartoonist Group is owned and managed by Sara Thaves. Sara is a cartoonist's legacy; her father created the comic strip *Frank and Ernest*, and her brother still produces it. She had already produced books with Cartoonist Group members Matt Wuerker (*The Cartoonist Group Inks Campaign '08*), Ann Telnaes (*Dick*), and Signe Wilkinson (*One Nation under Surveillance*). When I contacted her to ask about licenses and fees, Sara wondered whether I was the author of *Food Politics*. She had long wanted to showcase the food cartoons of artists in the group. Would I be interested? I most certainly would. I suspected that working with cartoons would be tremendous fun, as indeed it was. Sara and I talked. We met. This book is the result.

FOOD IS POLITICAL?

YES IT IS, as this book explains. Food is of extraordinary public interest. Everyone eats. In my writings about how politics influences what people eat, I approach the topic from the perspective of a public health nutritionist. Nutritionists teach individuals to make better food choices. But public health nutritionists take a broader view. We try to change the social, economic, and political environment so that it promotes the health and well-being of individuals. From a public health standpoint, food choices are not just personal decisions determined by cultural background, age, sex, peer group, education, or income. Food choices are also influenced by environmental factors. These include obvious ones such as advertising and marketing.

But they also include far more subtle influences such as product placement in supermarkets, portion size, price, and even how close at hand a food might be. The complexity and subtlety of these influences means that education alone is rarely enough to induce people to improve their diets. It works much better to change the food environment to make the healthier choice the easier—the default—choice.

This point, difficult to recognize as it may be, lies at the heart of current debates about food politics. Almost any aspect of food and nutrition—from science to policy, from farm to fork—generates controversy. Arguments about food issues derive from the complexity of foods and diets, and the uncertainty of the science linking diet to health. But the real reason for controversy is a difference in point of view. Dietary complexity and scientific uncertainty require interpretation. Interpretation depends on point of view. Point of view depends on cultural upbringing and value systems, but also on "stakeholder" position.

Because everyone eats, everyone has a vested interest—a stake—in how food is produced, sold, and consumed, and, therefore, in how food issues are interpreted. Stakeholders approach food issues from their own particular perspectives. Mine happens to be public health nutrition. I care about what it takes to promote health in the population as a whole, and I interpret both the science and the politics of food and nutrition from that point of view. From my public health standpoint, if government intervention in dietary choices improves health, it is a good thing to do.

I am well aware that not everyone shares this point of view. Americans particularly value personal autonomy, and many citizens believe that as long as their personal decisions do not directly harm others, the government should not interfere in what they choose to eat—even if those choices eventually make them ill and generate health care costs that must be borne by society.

This book is concerned with such views but also with those of government and the food industry. Government agencies issue dietary guidelines, support agricultural production, provide food assistance to the poor, and regulate such matters as food labeling, food advertising, food biotechnology, and food safety—all of which can affect the food choices of individuals. Although nearly every federal agency has something to do with food or nutrition, the two most important are the USDA and the Department of Health and Human Services (HHS). HHS is the parent agency of the Food and Drug Administration (FDA) and the Centers for Disease Control and Prevention (CDC). A separate agency, the Federal Trade Commission (FTC), regulates food advertising. These agencies act in their own interest or do the bidding of the White House or Congress, and they must respond to political pressures from constituents with widely varying needs, wants, demands, resources, and viewpoints. ▼

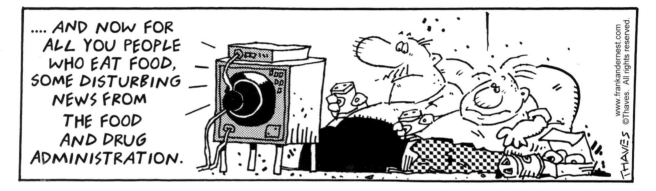

The food industry—a collective term for food and beverage companies and trade associations across the entire food system, from production to consumption—looks at food issues from a quite different perspective. Food is an enormous business that generates well over $1 trillion in annual sales in the United States alone. Food must be produced, processed, distributed, and prepared before it is eaten, each of these steps conducted by companies with special interests in what the government and nutritionists say about food choice. Advice to avoid one or another category of food can decrease sales or increase the cost of production, as can government regulations. Food companies and their trade associations recruit lobbyists to help persuade government agencies to avoid issuing advice or regulations that might reduce product sales.

Food, nutrition, and health advocacy organizations promote the nutritional health of the public and, sometimes, counter the actions of food companies or the actions or inactions of government. But their financial resources are nowhere near as extensive as those of food companies. Finally, and we are at last getting to the role of cartoonists, the media hold a stake in food and nutrition issues. Stories about controversial issues attract readers. Because controversy is much more interesting than its absence, reporters prefer it. Media attention—and that of cartoonists—tends to focus on the points of contention rather than on less newsworthy points of agreement. ▶

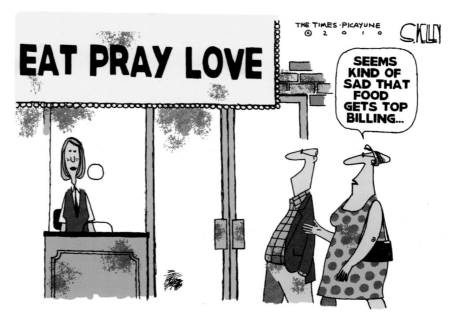

My food studies colleagues maintain that cultural background is the strongest influence on taste preferences and food choices—the proverbial "you are what you eat." But culture and taste can be modified by beliefs about food issues. Strongly held opinions about food derive, for example, from religion (it is wrong to eat shellfish or pork), ethics (it is wrong to kill animals for food), or philosophy (it is wrong to tamper with nature by genetically modifying foods). ▼

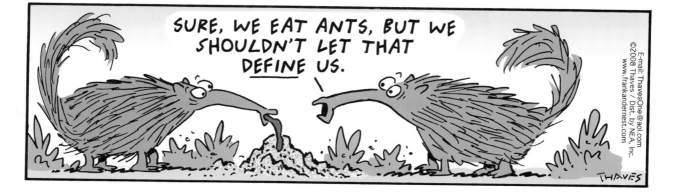

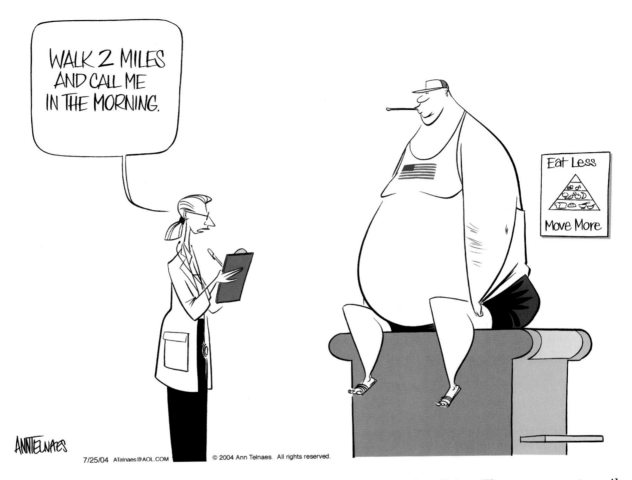

But this book is mainly concerned with opinions about food politics. These are most easily explained using obesity as an example. Obesity results from eating too many calories relative to those needed by the body. To lose weight, people must eat less, move more, or do both. Of these, eating less is more effective because it is difficult to work off excessive calorie intake through typical levels of physical activity. ▲

From my public health point of view, obesity is fostered by a food environment that encourages

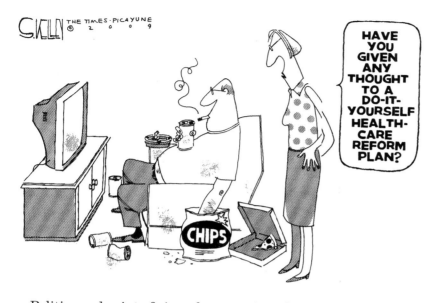

people to eat more often, in more places, and in larger amounts than is good for maintaining a healthy weight. As I explain in *Food Politics,* this environment evolved from the need of food companies to increase sales and to report quarterly growth to Wall Street in an enormously overabundant and competitive food marketplace. At this level of market competition, eating less is very bad for business. Hence: politics.

Politics and point of view also enter into discussions of what to do about obesity. If you believe that food choices are entirely a matter of personal responsibility, you are likely to believe that the food industry has no real influence over the diets of individuals and that the government has no business getting involved in anything having to do with your personal dietary decisions. If, on the other hand, you recognize that the food environment has a powerful influence on personal food choices, you may be willing to consider ways in which the government might put some limits on food industry marketing practices. ▲

For most of the topics discussed in this book, I state my public health viewpoint and describe the context in order to set the stage for the cartoonists' work. Cartoonists do more than entertain. They tap into the emotional core of complicated concepts and convey at a glance what might otherwise take pages to explain. When politics affects food choices, as it almost always does, cartoonists become astute commentators and social critics. Because food is such an intense focus of public discussion and connects to some of the most important issues facing societies today—and because the food industry acts in its own self-interest and government agencies act inconsistently—political cartoonists have plenty of material to work with.

ABOUT THE CARTOONS

"PLENTY TO WORK WITH" is why selecting the cartoons for this book proved exceptionally challenging. The Cartoonist Group includes about 50 members, many of them editorial cartoonists from nationally recognized newspapers, magazines, and Web sites who have been awarded Pulitzer and other impressive prizes (see About the Cartoonists, page 187). I was familiar with the work of several cartoonists in the group, but Sara Thaves started me off with a first mailing of about 300 cartoons and soon followed up with additional batches. By the time I begged her to stop, I had more than 1,000 cartoons to deal with, each better drawn, funnier, and more on target than the next. This was extraordinarily rich material—cartoon heaven—but I was going to have to pare them down to a publishable number.

How to choose? Sara wanted to include drawings by as many Cartoonist Group artists as possible. My Rodale Books editor, Alex Postman, wanted the drawings linked closely to the text. Rodale's book designers, Amy King and Mike Smith, wanted to be able to work with cartoons in a variety of sizes, shapes, and styles. With these criteria in mind, I began by sorting the cartoons into piles by topic, choosing the ones that best fit, and reluctantly rejecting wonderful drawings that did not work quite so well. Eventually, I met with the Rodale editorial team to thrash through the final selections.

I especially wanted this book to include cartoons that represent different points of view. Cartoonists often approach food topics from perspectives quite different from mine. For example, I tend to view overweight as a societal problem, but cartoonists do not always see it that way. They typically portray obesity by exaggerating body size. Such exaggerations can be offensive, and I would have preferred to keep such drawings to a minimum. But in the end, I decided to have my say in each chapter and let the cartoonists speak for themselves. Let the debates begin!

A NOTE TO READERS

I HAVE LONG BELIEVED that much of the excitement and enjoyment of studying food and nutrition derives from the complexity of the field and the many points of view that can be brought to bear on most aspects of research and practice in diet and health. Anyone interested in nutrition or food science—but also in history, sociology, anthropology, politics, biology, public health, medicine, law, or almost any other field of study—holds a legitimate stake in the issues debated in this book. Indeed, anyone who eats holds such a stake. Debates about food and nutrition are personal as well as political. For that reason, I think they are especially interesting, entertaining, and useful.

I hope that you will enjoy the different points of view and bring your own thoughts and opinions to food debates. I want these cartoons to inspire readers to become active in food politics and work toward a food system that is healthier for people and the planet. Join groups that are working on these issues. Vote with your fork! But food choices are also about politics. Exercise your democratic right as a citizen. Vote with your vote!

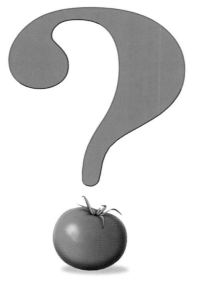

©2008 Clay Bennett.
Chattanooga Times Free Press BENNETT

1 The American Food System: From Farm to Table

FOOD IS POLITICAL BECAUSE PEOPLE HAVE WIDELY

varying interests in its production and consumption. As an eater, you might be concerned about the health effects of food, its cost, and whether you have adequate access to foods that you like and are good for you. If you are in the food business, your primary concern has to be about how to sell as much of your products as you possibly can at a profit. If you are a member of Congress, you might want to enact policies that please the majority of your constituents, but circumstances might require you to please some—contributors to your campaign funds, for example—more than others. And if you work for a government agency, even your best ideas about how to improve the food system will be constrained by the political considerations of the party in power.

The food industry is vast. It encompasses everyone who owns or works in agriculture (animal and plant), product manufacture, restaurants, institutional food service, retail stores, and factories that make farm machines and fertilizers, as well as people engaged in the transportation, storage, and insurance businesses that support such enterprises. ▼

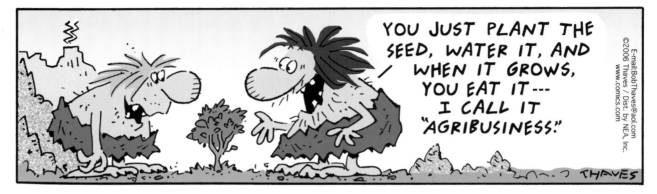

This means that any labor, safety, advertising, or labeling regulation; any program of farm support or food assistance; any law governing taxes, food aid, immigration, or international trade; and any federal dietary recommendation has the potential to affect the sales, income, and livelihoods of anyone involved.

THE US AGRICULTURAL SYSTEM

THE CURRENT FOOD SYSTEM in the United States is largely based on industrial agriculture—CAFOs (confined animal feeding operations) and enormous farms—and supermarket aisles overflowing with snacks, candies, cookies, sodas, and sugary foods that bear little resemblance to the plants, crops, or animals from which they were derived. This system is highly efficient and provides an abundance of foods from which to choose at relatively low cost, but with unfortunate consequences for health and the environment, especially when companies cut corners on labor and safety practices. Pressures to keep wages low, for example, mean that only immigrants are willing to do farm labor. Immigrants have always done work that nobody else wants to do, and farm labor is the most recent example. One unintended consequence of policies that restrict immigration is to reduce the supply of agricultural workers. ▼ ▶

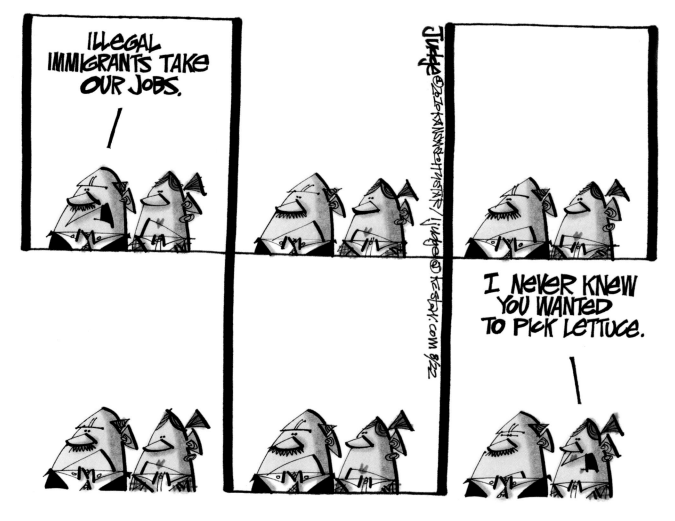

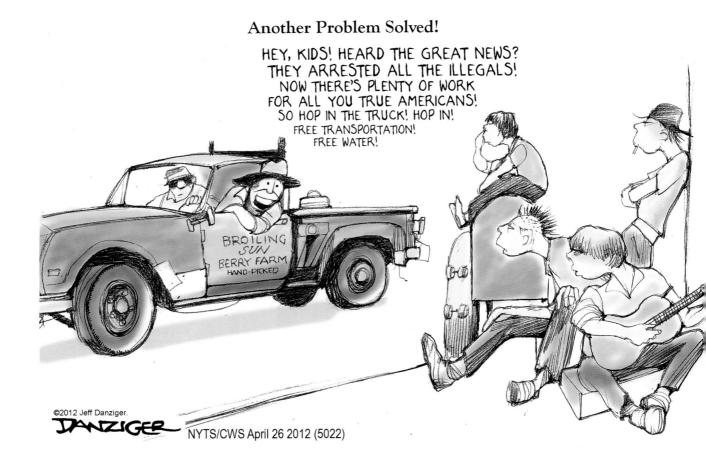

Federal dietary guidelines may encourage consumption of fruits and vegetables, but federal subsidies go almost exclusively to the growers of food commodities such as corn and soybeans. These crops are grown mainly for animal feed. In contrast, the USDA has historically considered fruits and vegetables to be "specialty" crops, undeserving of much in the way of federal support. Although this support system began in the 1930s as a means to ensure enough food for Americans and a reasonable living for small farmers, farms got bigger over the years. The invention of new machines led to greater efficiency and meant that fewer workers were needed. ▼

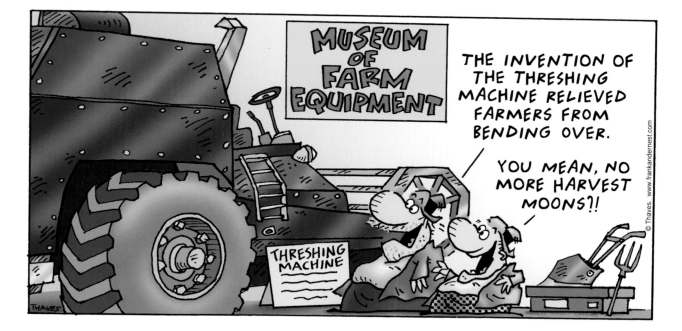

Consolidation of agricultural production also led to greater efficiency. These changes resulted in federal subsidies going to larger and richer farms.

Congress determines subsidies and other forms of agricultural support through long, complicated, and expensive farm bills, renegotiated about every five years. The 2008 farm bill, for example, cost taxpayers about $20 billion a year for direct payments, conservation, and insurance support programs. Direct payments were by far the most contentious form of agricultural support. The bill authorized payments to the owners of the largest farms, many of them wealthy landowners who live in cities, rent out the land, never set foot on the farms, and simply collect the checks. ▼

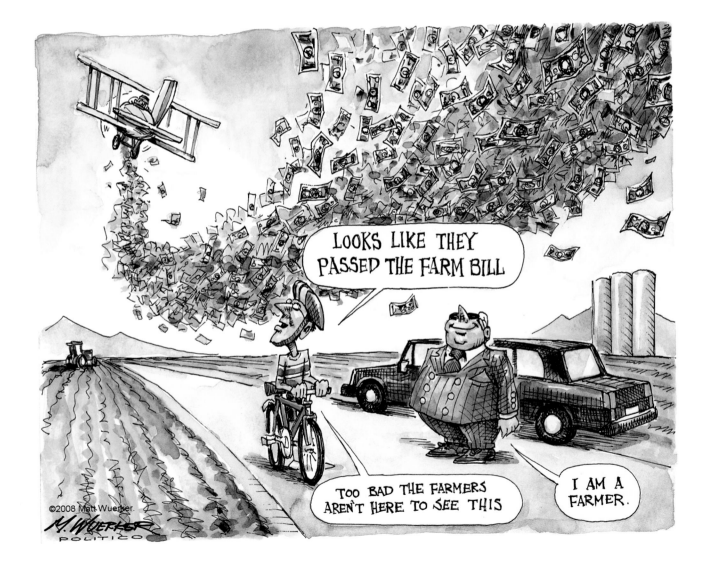

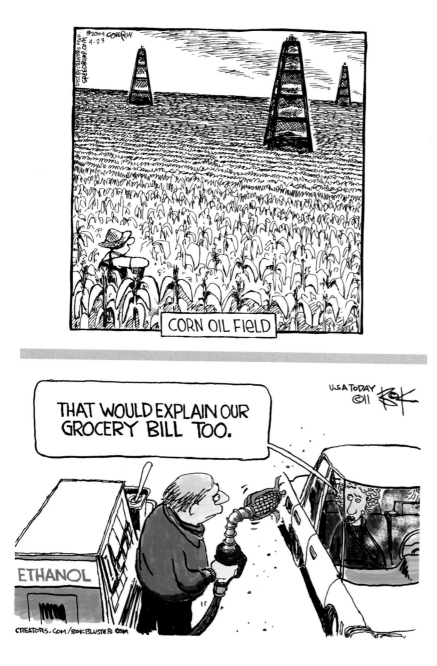

CORN OIL FIELD

THAT WOULD EXPLAIN OUR GROCERY BILL TOO.

ETHANOL

In 2005 and 2007, Congress passed energy policy acts that required increasing percentages of ethanol to be mixed with gasoline. Farmers quickly began diverting corn crops from animal feed to ethanol production. By 2012, more than 40 percent of US corn was used to produce ethanol. Given the oil and gas used to produce fertilizer and to plant and harvest crops, it is debatable whether ethanol actually adds to our energy supply. But one result of the diversion is not debatable: Using corn to produce biofuels drives up food prices. This happened in the United States and also, as I explain in the next chapter, throughout the world. ◄ ◄

FOOD SYSTEM POLITICS

THE HISTORY OF AGRICULTURE policy in the United States is one of increasing concentration and consolidation, with big driving out small in the name of efficiency. It is also one of cozy relations between corporate agriculture, Congress, and the USDA. For decades, representatives from farm states ran congressional agriculture and agricultural appropriations committees, and the USDA worked closely with agribusiness to promote larger and more efficient production. Food product manufacturers also benefited from this system, especially at the state level. In the wake of antiobesity lawsuits against McDonald's in the early 2000s, states began to introduce laws to protect food companies from such "frivolous" suits. More than 20 states passed "cheeseburger"

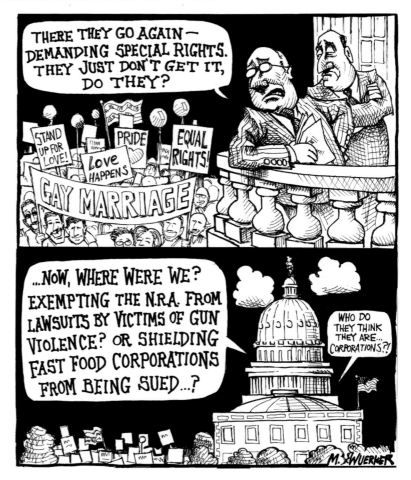

bills protecting restaurants and food product companies from obesity lawsuits, and Congress introduced legislation to limit such lawsuits in state courts. Such actions conveyed the impression that Congress, the USDA, and agribusiness had the same pro-business goals. ▲

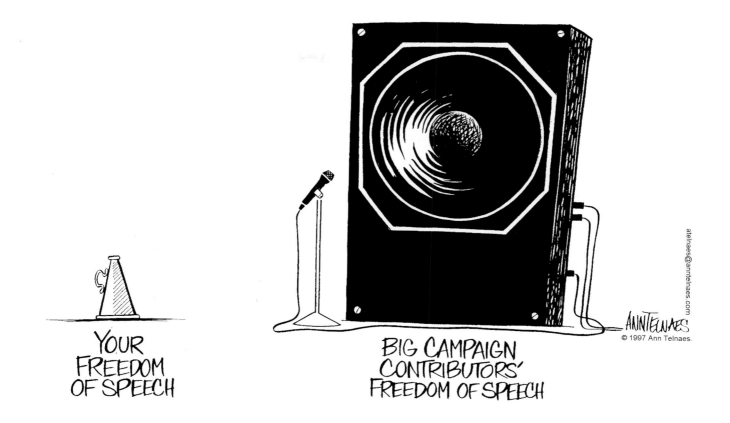

YOUR FREEDOM OF SPEECH

BIG CAMPAIGN CONTRIBUTORS' FREEDOM OF SPEECH

ANNTELNAES

atelnaes@anntelnaes.com

© 1997 Ann Telnaes.

In 2010, the Supreme Court ruled that the First Amendment to the US Constitution—freedom of speech—allowed corporations and private groups to donate as much money as they liked to candidates for election. Corporations, however, have far greater resources than most food advocacy groups. ▲

This case, *Citizens United v. Federal Election Commission,* opened the floodgates to unlimited campaign contributions through super PACs, political action committees able to accept anonymous contributions from food and agriculture corporations through a new loophole: money funneled through nonprofit groups. The influx of this anonymous "dark money" reinforced the suspicion that congressional candidates are for sale to the highest bidders. ▼

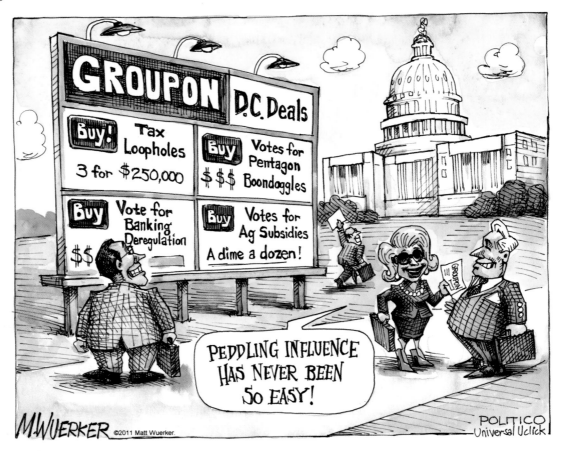

What seem to be simple decisions about food issues that affect public health are instead influenced by the need for candidates to raise money to run for office. That money influences federal policy seems self-evident but turns out to be difficult to prove, thereby leaving the question open to speculation and opinion. Opinions, as always, depend on point of view. But one unarguable result of unlimited campaign spending is that Congress often *appears* to be more concerned with the health of corporations than with the health of the public.

TODAY'S FOOD MARKETING ENVIRONMENT

THE PREVALENCE OF OBESITY in the United States began to rise sharply starting in the early 1980s. Since then, our food environment has changed in ways that encourage eating in more places, with greater frequency, and in much larger portions. In part, these changes in society happened as a result of the increasingly frantic pace of modern life. ▼

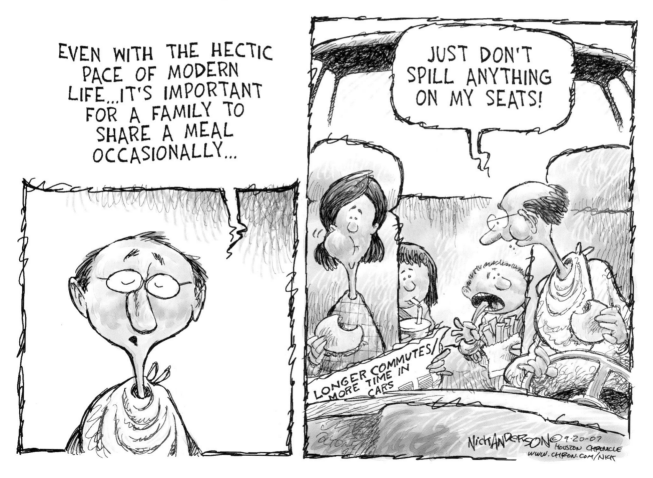

But they also occurred as a result of changes in agricultural and investment policies that forced food companies to become more competitive. Through the 1960s, federal agricultural policy aimed to keep prices high by reducing the supply of commodities. The USDA paid growers of commodity crops to let land lie fallow. But beginning in the 1970s, Congress removed such restrictions and began rewarding farmers for growing as much food as they could fit

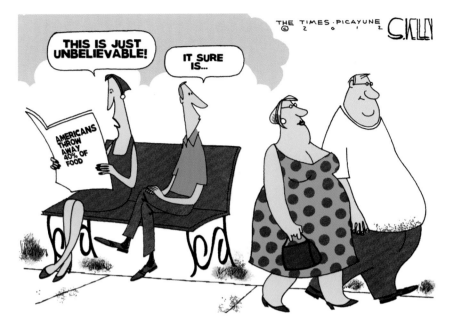

onto their land. The number of calories available in the food supply—available but not necessarily consumed—rose from about 3,200 per day per capita in 1980 to 3,900 by the year 2000. Calorie availability is calculated on the basis of all food produced in the United States, plus food that is imported, minus food exports. Per capita includes men, women, children, and tiny babies. Overall, 3,900 calories a day is roughly twice the average need of the population. Even if a great deal of food is wasted, calories are still available in great excess. ▲

The overabundance of calories forces the food industry to be highly competitive, but other changes in the early 1980s required even more competition. Shareholders began to pressure corporations to reward them with higher immediate returns on investment. Food companies not only had to compete for sales against 3,900 calories a day, but now had to *increase* sales and report growth in profits to Wall Street every 90 days. Competitive pressures forced food companies to consolidate, to become larger and more efficient, to seek new markets, and to expand existing markets. Fast-food places proliferated. The mere presence of fast-food places selling cheap, high-calorie foods, backed

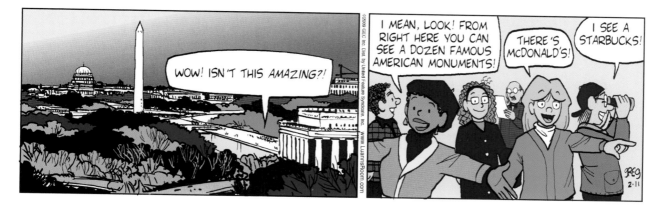

up by enormous amounts of advertising, is all it takes to induce customers to buy products and eat more than they should. ▲

Vending machines were installed in schools. Companies began to market foods in places where food had never been sold in the past: bookstores, libraries, and stores selling clothing, business supplies, cosmetics, or drugs. And restaurants began serving foods in larger and larger portions. ▼

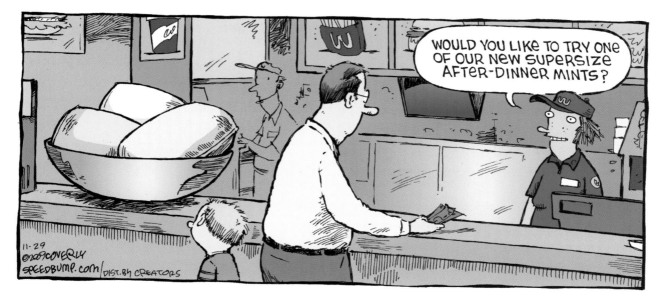

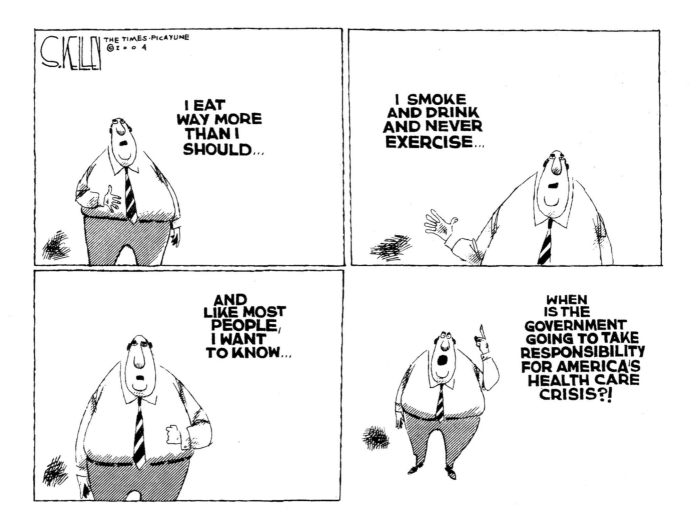

Today, it has become socially acceptable to eat in more places, more frequently, and in much larger amounts. Fast food and sodas have become ubiquitous parts of the American landscape. Eating more is good for business. Eating less is not. The result: Overeating is not nearly so much a problem of weak character as an unavoidable response to today's "eat more" food environment.

Former FDA Commissioner David Kessler, MD, argues in *The End of Overeating* (Rodale, 2009)

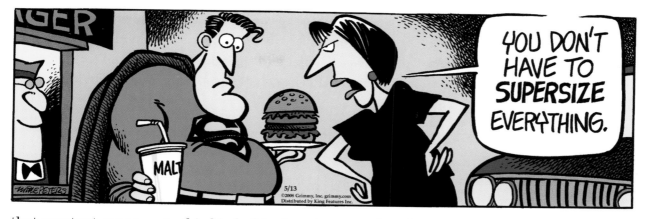

that constant exposure to this kind of food environment has driven people to desire high-calorie fast foods, snacks, and beverages, and to become "conditioned overeaters." The current food environment induces people to eat more food than they need or necessarily want, not least because "eat more" stimuli are largely invisible or not consciously perceived. But wait. Before blaming the food industry and government, shouldn't individuals bear the ultimate responsibility for making healthier choices regardless of the environment? ◄ ▲

Should educators focus on teaching people to make healthier choices? Or would they do better if they taught coping strategies for dealing with the not-so-obvious marketing efforts of food companies, supermarkets, and restaurants? ▼

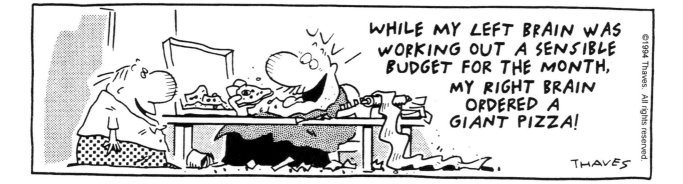

I sometimes like to ask: What industries benefit if people make healthier dietary choices? Not the food industry, which needs people to eat more, not less. Not the health care industry, which gets paid for treatment procedures and drugs. Not the diet or drug industries. What all this means is that dealing with the "eat more" food environment is a challenge—not only for individuals, but also for society. ▼ ▶

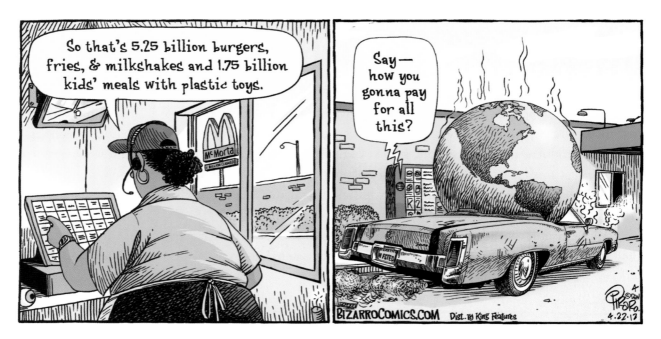

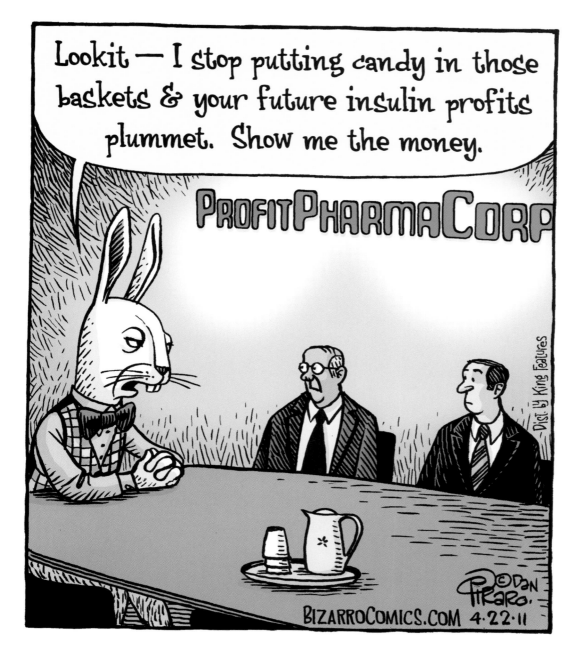

2 Why Food Production Matters: Hunger and Its Consequences

THE WORLD PRODUCES AN ABUNDANCE OF FOOD, more than enough to meet the needs of its more than six billion people. But food is distributed unequally. Not everyone has enough resources to obtain adequate food on a reliable basis. In public health terms, such people lack "food security." Whether or not food insecurity causes people to go hungry, it poses a difficult problem for societies and governments.

HUNGER IN AMERICA

ALTHOUGH FOOD IN AMERICA is abundant, not everyone has equal access to it. In the 1960s, the discovery of widespread malnutrition in rural areas of the South shocked the nation and led President Lyndon Johnson to declare war on poverty. Congress enacted food assistance programs such as food stamps. These helped. The prevalence of malnutrition declined.

Beginning in the 1980s, however, reductions in government expenditures, rising inflation, and losses in higher paying jobs widened the income gap. Government agencies began to document increasing levels of food insecurity. Today, USDA economists say that nearly 15 percent of US households are food insecure, with 5 percent seriously so. The least secure segments of the population are households with children headed by single women, especially those black or Hispanic. Economists estimate that 22 percent of American children live in homes with incomes below the poverty line. Hunger, they conclude, still exists in America.▼

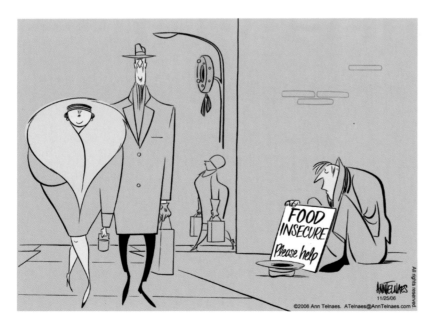

FOOD INSECURE Please help

Welfare policies dating back to the English Poor Laws of the 16th century reveal that societies have always struggled to balance humanitarian goals—providing food to the hungry—against concerns about the cost of such assistance and fears of inducing dependency in recipients. Even today, food assistance policies tread a fine line between providing enough food to keep people from starving or taking to the streets, but not giving them so much that they can live comfortably.

For many out-of-work and out-of-luck Americans, some formerly in the middle class, having to balance food purchases against other necessities has become a normal part of daily existence. ▶

When Congress enacted food stamp legislation, it made the program an entitlement. Anyone who met income limitations could obtain benefits. The program is now called the Supplemental Nutrition Assistance Program (SNAP) in recognition that participants use Electronic Benefit Transfer (EBT) cards rather than stamps to purchase food. In 2012, the declining economy and increasing rates of unemployment drove a record-setting 46.6 million Americans—many of them working for low wages and half of them children—to obtain SNAP benefits. Although the average benefit was only about $135 per month, the total cost to taxpayers was $75 billion that year. ▶

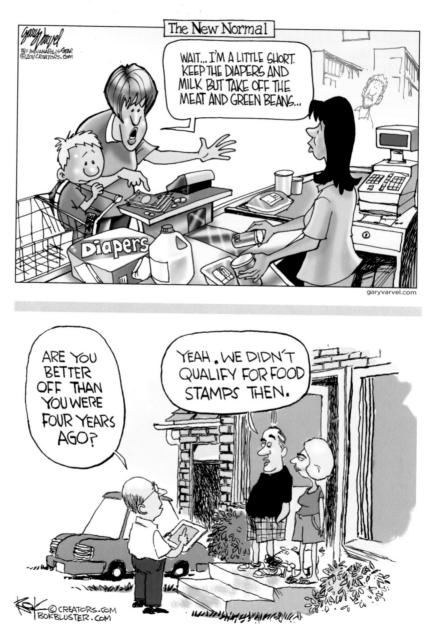

If millions of Americans do not have enough food for lack of jobs or other resources, shouldn't governments expand welfare and food assistance benefits to make sure that no adult or child goes hungry? Those opposed to current food assistance policies argue that food insecurity is more a result of unwillingness to work and erosion of family values than of failings in society. ▼

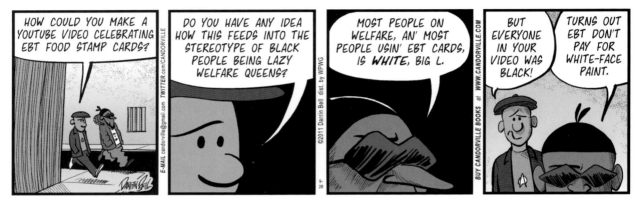

Critics of federal food assistance complain that the programs cost too much, are beset by fraud, and mostly encourage dependency. ▶

The private sector, they say, is better equipped to feed the poor. This view has led to the creation of an enormous enterprise devoted to food banks, soup kitchens, and other sources of charitable food. Whether these can possibly meet the needs of

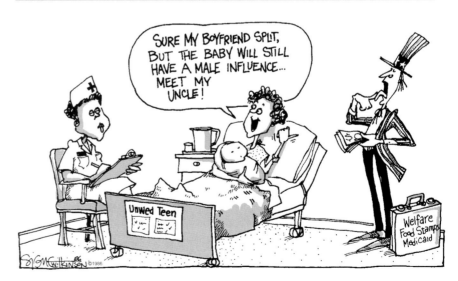

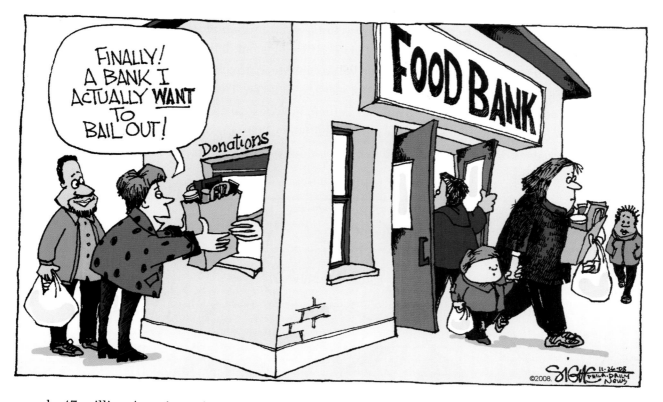

nearly 47 million Americans is arguable, but one effect is well established: Giving food to the poor makes donors feel good about themselves. ▲

Arguments about food assistance must deal with one of the great ironies of hunger in America. The highest prevalence of overweight and obesity is observed among the poor. Researchers examining the apparent paradox of hunger in the land of plenty note that food insecurity is a significant predictor of overweight, particularly in low-income groups. They explain the paradox as an effect of inadequate resources. SNAP benefits, for example, are meant to be supplemental and typically run out after two or three weeks, leading recipients to depend on the cheapest sources of calories—the snacks, fast food, and sugar-sweetened sodas pejoratively called "junk foods" or, more politely, "foods of minimal nutritional value."

Whether it is acceptable in so rich a country to have 22 million children living in poverty and reliant on SNAP benefits depends on point of view. At issue is not only how to reduce the disparities in income, education, health, and cultural values between the haves and have-nots, but also whether it is necessary for our American democracy to do so. I would argue yes. Others might disagree. Because this argument depends on values, how best to end hunger in America becomes a matter of politics. As is the case with many food issues, the question of whether government assistance increases dependency depends on who you are. The poor are not alone in enjoying the benefits of government largesse. ▼▶

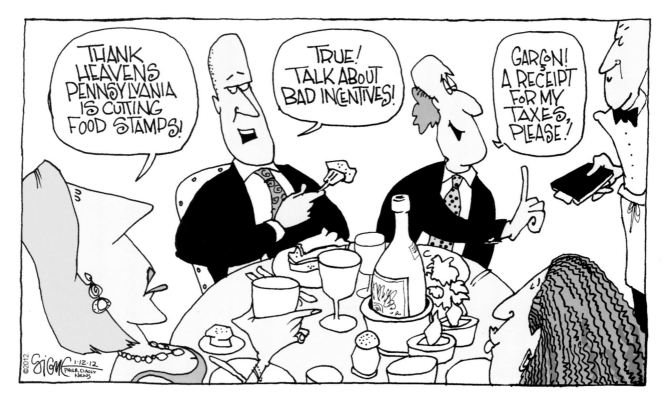

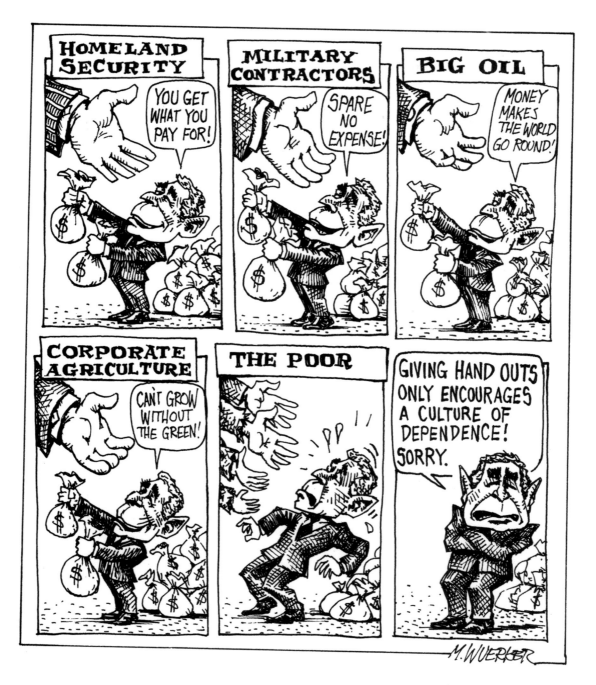

HUNGER IN THE WORLD

THE FOOD AND Agriculture Organization of the United Nations estimates that 870 million people, most of them young children in the developing world, do not have enough to eat or lack a reliable source of food from day to day. As a result, they are hungry, become malnourished, and may die prematurely. This tragedy, almost entirely preventable, has little to do with food production. Most countries produce or import more than enough food for their populations, but whether they can continue to do so in the face of future population growth remains to be seen. ▶▶

At the moment, world hunger and starvation have everything to do with politics. Political conflict, insufficient responses to natural disasters, corrupt political institutions,

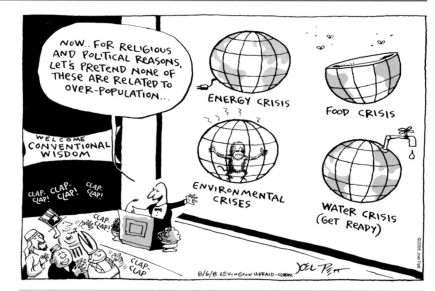

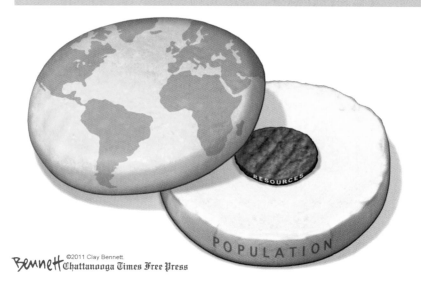

and inequalities in income and education constitute what public health practitioners call the "root" causes of hunger and malnutrition. ▼

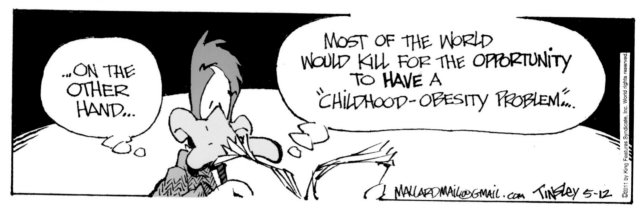

Here, too, ironies abound. As world economies improve, some segments of their populations can afford to eat better and want to eat the way Americans do. Just as we do, they buy junk foods higher in calories, gain weight, and become obese. As the economies of developing countries improve, the number of obese people in the world rises to equal or exceed the number considered food insecure. ▶

Another irony derives from the results of congressional insistence that gasoline be

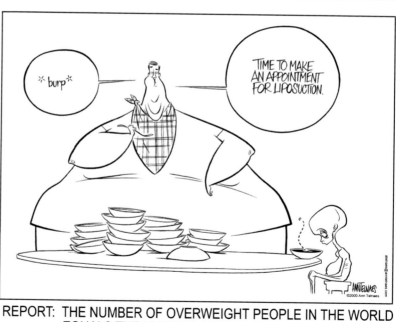

REPORT: THE NUMBER OF OVERWEIGHT PEOPLE IN THE WORLD EQUALS THE NUMBER OF MALNOURISHED PEOPLE.

mixed with ethanol. As I noted in Chapter 1, US farmers responded to congressional incentives by planting corn and soybeans for biofuels. Economists consider the use of food crops for fuel to be the single most important reason for the recent sharp rise in worldwide food prices and worldwide hunger. Millions of people suddenly could not afford to buy the food they need. ▶ ▶

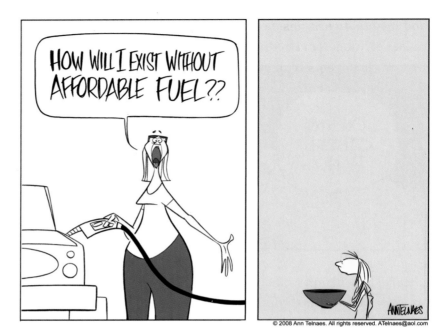

In many countries, thousands of desperate people took to the streets to demand that their governments provide food at prices they could afford. ▶ ▶

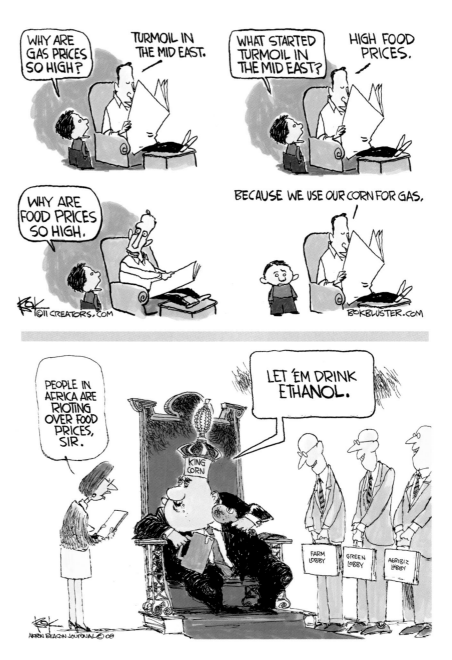

FOOD IN INTERNATIONAL RELATIONS

FOOD INSECURITY IN developing countries made worse by biofuel-induced high prices has led to a worldwide crisis. The governments of developing countries complain—with considerable justification—that richer countries ignore their problems except when it advances the donors' own self-interest. ▼

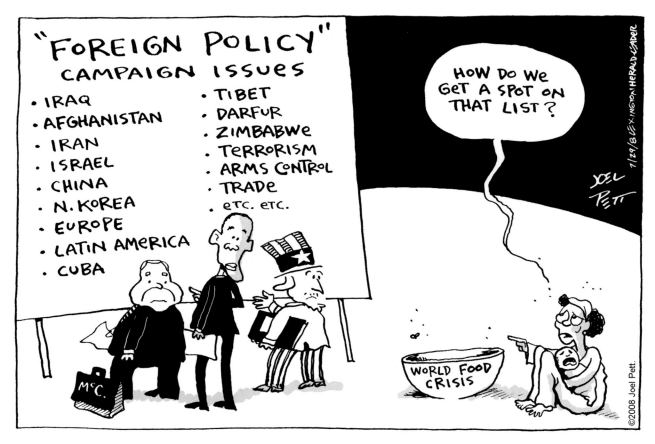

Food aid has long been used to promote the foreign policy of the United States. The government buys surplus agricultural products and donates or sells them at low cost to foreign countries to help governments we favor or to create alliances with those we don't. Because the United States is so rich a country, the governments of poorer countries may perceive us as ungenerous or acting more in our own self-interest than as responding to the real needs of their populations. They have a point. Aid policies are often designed to reward American companies or dispose of agricultural surpluses or discarded foods, rather than to help countries develop their own agricultural self-sufficiency. ▲

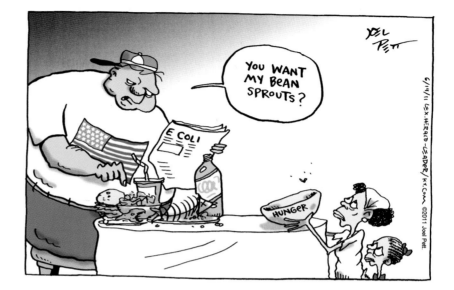

In recent years, the use—or misuse—of food aid has become especially contentious when aimed at the populations of countries whose governments are perceived as hostile to our interests. In places rife with political violence, food becomes unavailable to refugees fleeing the conflict and to people trapped in cities under siege. Fighting depletes food stocks and disrupts food supply chains. Rising prices put foods beyond the reach of people caught in conflict. In Libya in 2011, in the midst of the Arab Spring, groups rallied to oppose its dictatorial government. The US government authorized large shipments of vegetable oil and pinto beans to help those who had fled the country. But this did little to eliminate the food crisis brought on, in part, by the United States' own fuel policies. ▶

North Korea is another example. Since the mid-1990s, North Korea has suffered from chronic food shortages, reportedly causing the death by starvation of 5 to 10 percent of its population. Food aid donated by China, South Korea, and the United States helped to relieve this crisis. From 1995 through 2008, Americans provided North Korea with more than half a billion dollars in food aid. But

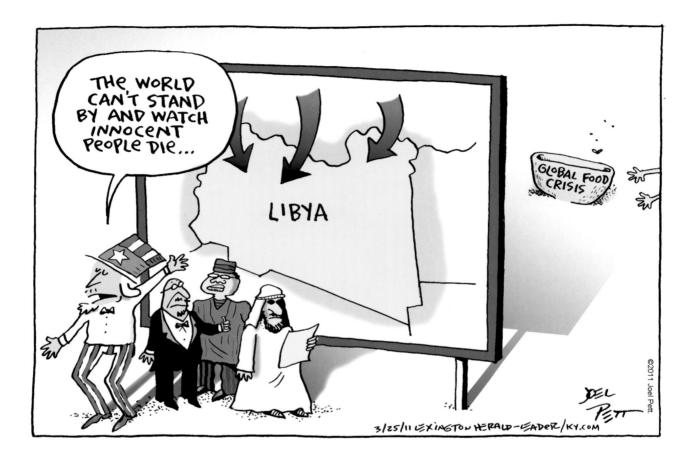

when North Korea launched a long-range missile program, the US government stopped donations. In 2011, North Korea called on international donors to provide more food, and the United Nations issued an appeal for assistance. When North Korea said it would end its missile program and nuclear testing, the US government reinstated food aid but issued a warning that any breach in the moratorium would put further aid at risk.

Providing food aid to North Korea poses delicate political problems for the United States. The North Korean government imposes restrictive policies on its people and, as often happens, allows food aid to be diverted for resale in private markets. But without food aid, millions may starve. Should the United States provide food aid to North Korea? And if so, should aid be conditional on guarantees of international security or human rights? And does its nutritional quality matter? ▼

The role of food in international relations points out a key theme of this book: Food provides an accessible entry point into discussions of the most important issues facing the world today. Cartoonists track such issues closely for two reasons: the intrinsic importance of the issues and the enormous public interest in them.

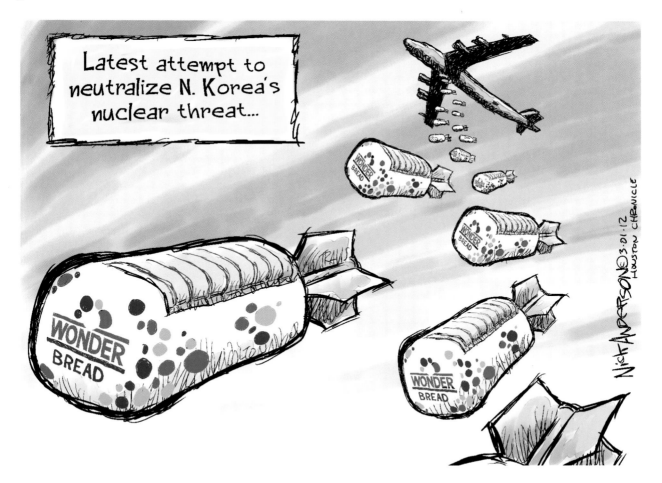

3

Why Food Production Matters: Obesity and What to Do about It

TO PUBLIC HEALTH PROFESSIONALS, THE rising prevalence of obesity in the United States and elsewhere constitutes a health challenge of crisis proportions. ▶

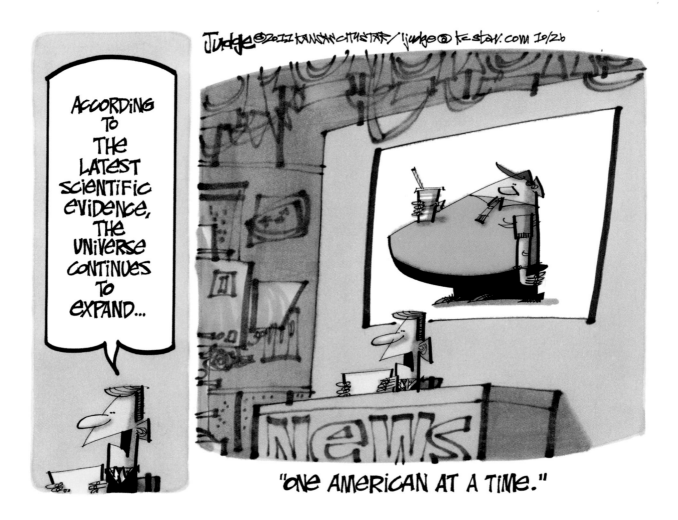

"ONE AMERICAN AT A TIME."

Not every overweight person will develop a chronic disease, but obesity makes type 2 diabetes, heart disease, and other problems much more likely to occur.

Obesity would seem to be the most personal of health problems, but it is highly political. Why? People differ in beliefs about its cause, whether anything needs to be done about it, and, if so, what.

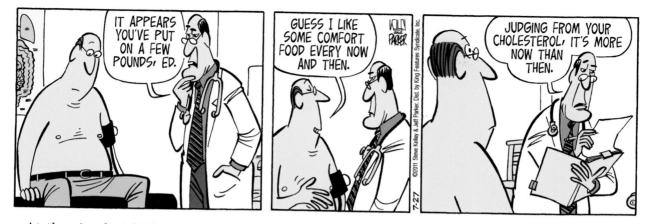

At the simplest biological level, gaining weight is the result of consuming too many calories for those expended. We must eat to survive. Hunger makes us want to eat. Food is delicious and one of life's greatest pleasures, one repeated several times a day. Food is easily accessible, and today's society encourages indulgence. ▼

But why do some people seem to gain weight more easily than others? Genetics is certainly a factor, but genetics has not had time to change since Americans began to put on weight in the 1980s.

What did change was the food environment. Beginning in the early 1980s, food became more widely available. Fast-food places proliferated. The sizes of food portions increased. People began to eat outside the home more often and to snack more frequently. This is why obesity poses a

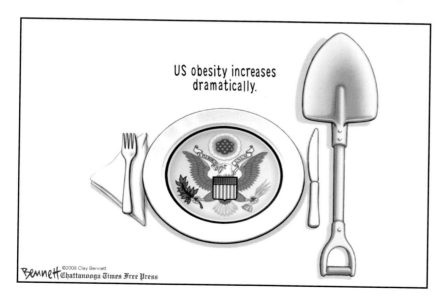

particular challenge to cartoonists. They can quickly draw enormous bellies to illustrate the personal factors that contribute to obesity, but they find the environmental influences more difficult to characterize. ▼

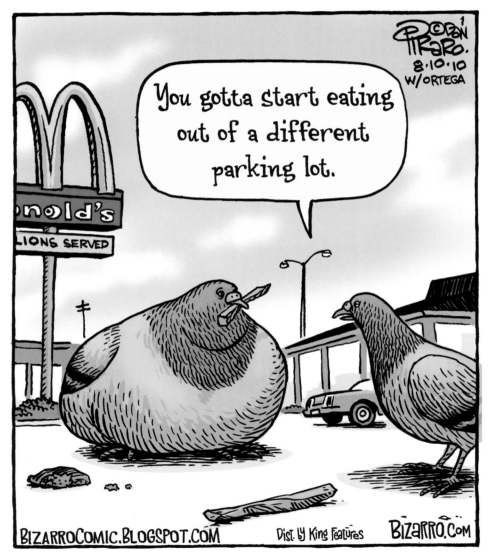

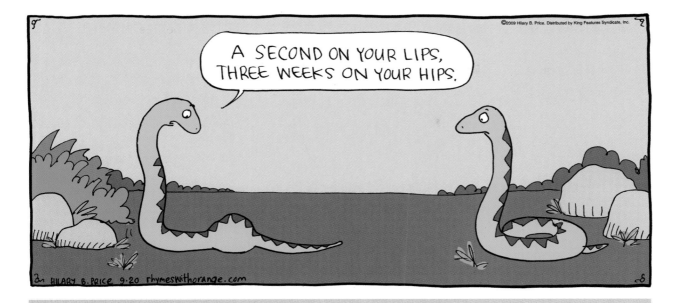

Because trends in the food environment contributed to greater calorie intake, people who used to be able to maintain their body weight could no longer do so. As more people put on pounds, overweight became the norm. ▲

Americans on average have gained 20 pounds or more since the early 1960s, but heights have increased by an inch or less. Any level of overweight can raise the risk of disease in susceptible people, but mortality rates increase most in the extremely overweight. ▶

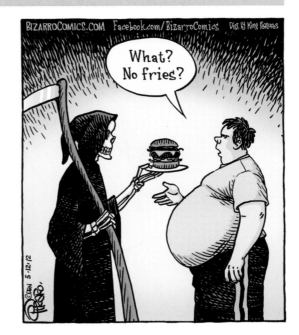

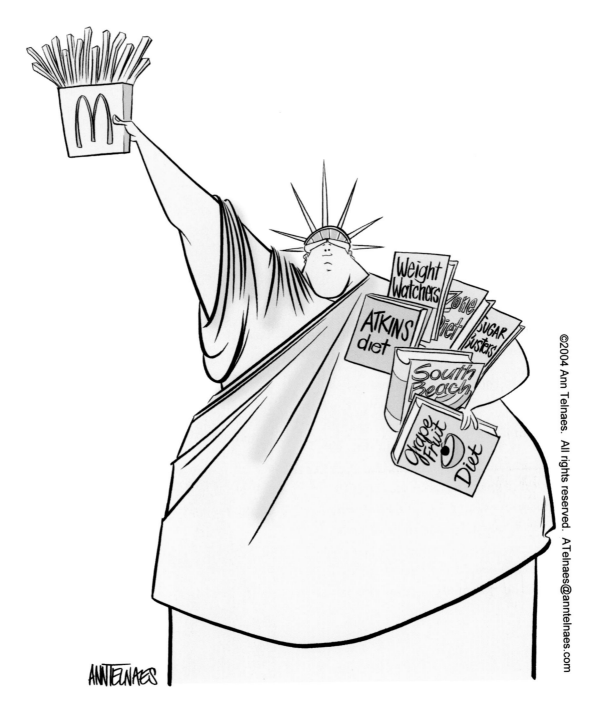

EAT LESS

TO PREVENT OBESITY, people must reduce calorie intake ("eat less"), preferably by eating more healthfully ("eat better"), or they must increase calorie expenditure ("move more"). Doing all three works best. But these actions are exceedingly difficult for most people to manage in today's food marketing environment.

Eating less, as I've mentioned, may be bad for food sales, but trying to help people eat less is very good for the diet industry. Americans spend about $60 billion a year on diet books, plans, programs, pills, and weight loss surgery. ◄

Dieting, however, is rarely effective for long-term weight loss. Most people who lose weight regain it over time, mainly because dieting fights physiology. Although a great many hormones and factors are involved in regulation of hunger, satiety, and body weight, nearly all of them stimulate people to eat; hardly any tell you when to stop. Scientists evoke evolutionary explanations for this imbalance—humans evolved from populations who had to hunt or gather. When food intake drops below the amount required for physiological needs, metabolism slows to conserve energy and you need fewer calories. Once you do lose weight, you need even fewer calories to maintain your smaller body size. Dieters must counter their own physiology as well as the "eat more" food environment. Under these circumstances, personal responsibility doesn't stand a chance. ▼

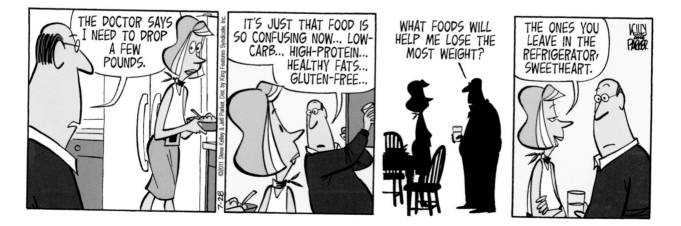

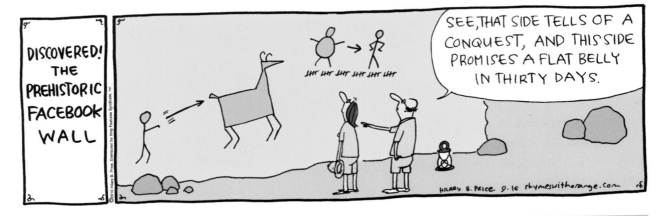

Dieting to lose weight is as old as recorded history. Hippocrates discussed diets and dieting in the pre-Christian era, and to-day's diet books are perennial bestsellers. ▲

Dieting may fight physiology, but it also fights human nature. We love to eat, and dieting is anything but fun. Dieters are always looking for easy ways to eat less without having to endure deprivation. ▶

How to "eat better" is so important that it gets its own chapter (Chapter 4). For now, let's consider the activity side of maintaining weight.

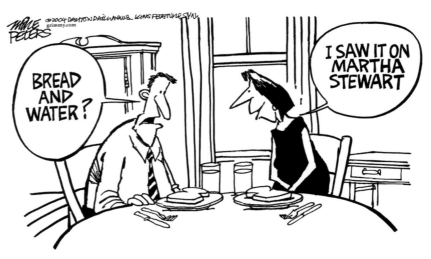

MOVE MORE

PHYSICAL ACTIVITY—the normal moving around that people do during daily life and work, as well as the more intense actions involved in deliberate exercise—is well established to promote good health. Activity strengthens muscles, reduces risk factors for chronic disease, and feels good. It also helps maintain body weight. The amount of activity needed to obtain benefits is uncertain, but the standard recommendation is for about a half hour of moderate or vigorous exercise on most days. This amount, however, is far more than most people are able or want to do. ▼

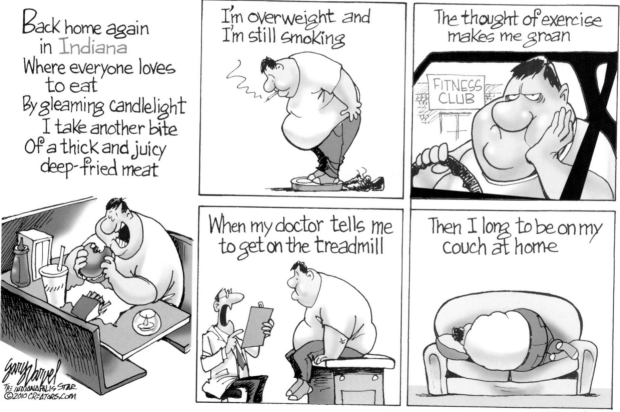

garyvarvel.com

Many factors in modern society encourage inactivity, television most of all. Since its invention, researchers have been interested in how TV affects the eating habits of viewers. Watching TV is a sedentary behavior that requires little or no calorie expenditure. Many programs are accompanied by repeated commercials for high-calorie junk foods and soft drinks, and people tend to eat precisely those foods while watching TV. ▶

A demonstrably effective way to avoid putting on excess pounds is to turn off the TV. But being a "couch potato" is so much a part of American life that it is difficult to find effective ways to discourage this behavior. ▶ ▶

Automobiles, elevators, escalators, computers, and long workdays make it increasingly difficult for people to include physical activity—even

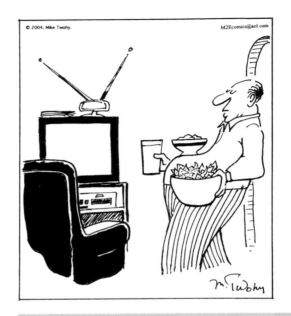

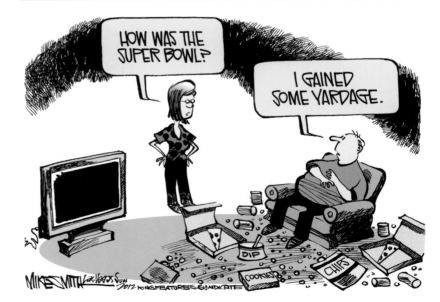

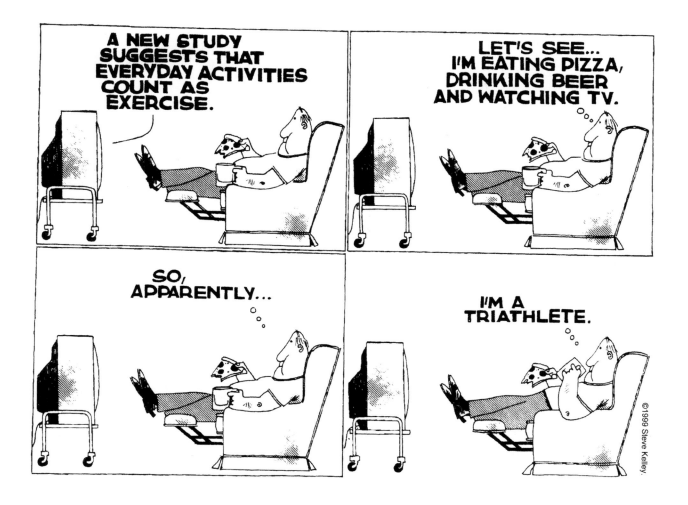

walking or climbing stairs—into daily lives. Being active is demonstrably good for health. Physical activity tunes up metabolism, strengthens muscles, reduces body fat, and helps prevent obesity and its related chronic diseases. Being active does not require joining a gym. Any physical activity counts: walking, climbing stairs, bicycling, dancing, gardening, doing housework—any-

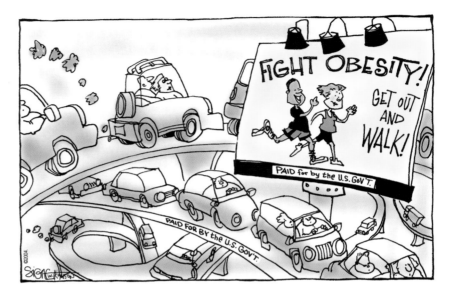

thing that gets your body moving. Some physical activity is better than none. More is better than less. But in today's environment, it's just as easy to find reasons not to move as it is to overeat. ▲ ▼

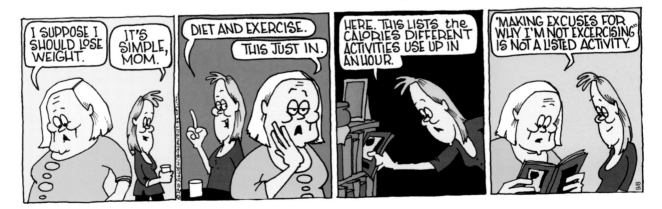

SHOULD THE GOVERNMENT INTERVENE?

A FREQUENT ARGUMENT against government intervention is that overweight does no harm to anyone other than the individual concerned. ▼

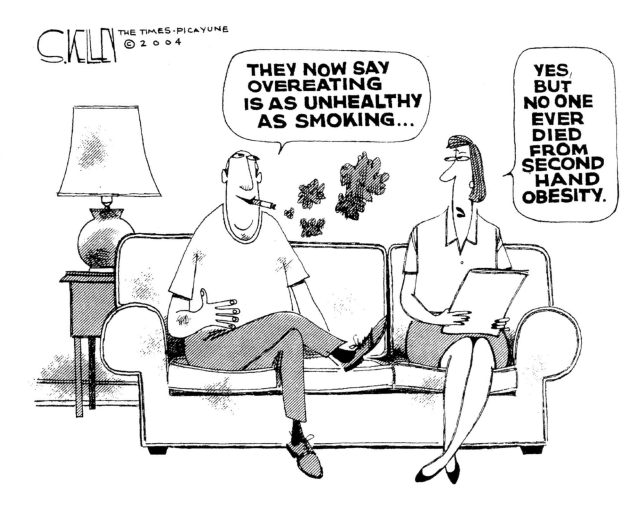

But economists argue that obesity generates costs beyond those to overweight individuals. They estimate the cost to society—in health care and lost productivity—as close to $190 billion per year. Figures like this induce government agencies to take action. The military, for example, complains that obesity is the principal reason why volunteers do not meet its physical fitness and weight requirements. It views the food environment as a national security threat equivalent to that of terrorism. ▼

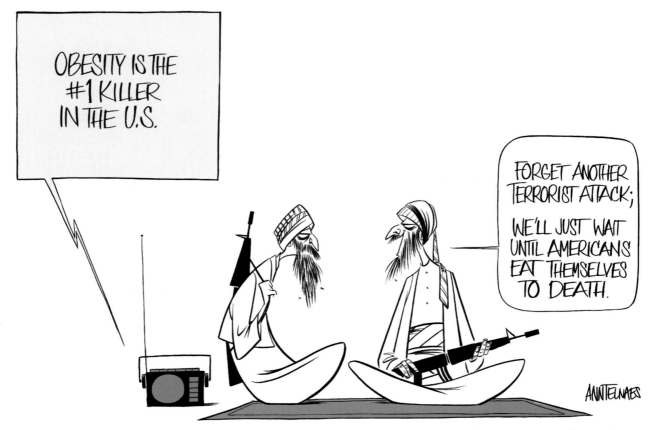

In 2010, Michelle Obama launched the nationwide campaign "Let's Move," with an ambitious agenda: to reverse childhood obesity within a generation. I found it thrilling that no less than the First Lady of the United States had become interested in my kind of public health issues. Others, who believe that the government should stay out of matters involving personal dietary choices, were less delighted, putting obesity in the same controversial category as climate change. ▶▶

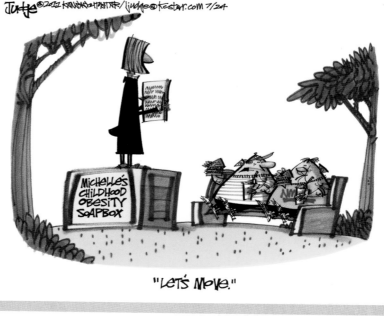

"Let's move."

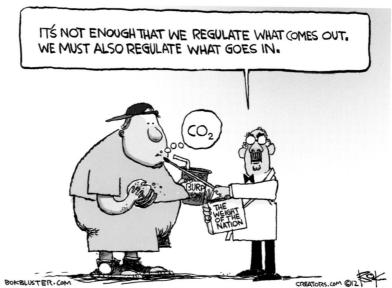

4 What Are We Supposed to Eat?

WHAT DOES "EAT BETTER" MEAN, EXACTLY? AS we've seen, people who do not have enough to eat are hungry and, in the most extreme situation, die of starvation. But those who eat too much gain weight and are more likely to develop conditions related to obesity and poor diets—coronary heart disease, cancer, diabetes, and stroke—that are now leading causes of death and disability in most world populations. Throughout human history, people have eaten foods available locally and through trade to meet nutritional needs. Widely different traditional dietary patterns and practices promote health and longevity, and it ought to be possible to enjoy the pleasures of food and eat healthfully at the same time. But it doesn't always appear that way. Current dietary advice can feel as though food has been transformed from the delicious, satisfying, and pleasurable to the frightening, coercive, and medicinal. ▶ ▶

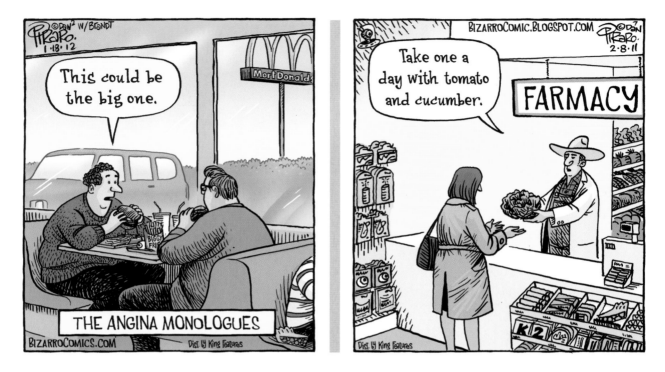

In the United States, the USDA has issued dietary advice to the public for nearly a century. Until the mid-1970s, USDA nutritionists advised people to eat a variety of foods every day from different groups—dairy, meat, fruits and vegetables, and cereals, and sometimes fats and sweets—to prevent nutrient deficiencies. Such advice elicited little controversy. As long as its purpose was to encourage eating more of American agricultural products, food companies were happy with it.

After World War II, disease patterns shifted. Nutrient deficiencies declined and were replaced by chronic diseases related to obesity and poor diets. It became necessary to advise eating less of foods containing nutritional factors that raised disease risks—saturated fat, cholesterol, sugar, salt, and alcohol—and eating less in general to balance calories. "Eat less" advice conflicts with the food industry's sales imperatives. It also conflicts with the USDA's mission to promote greater consumption of American agricultural products. Once "eat less" and "eat better" advice replaced advice to "eat more," the history of USDA food guides became one of ongoing controversy.

WHAT THE GOVERNMENT SAYS: PYRAMIDS

IN THE EARLY 1980s, USDA nutritionists began work on a food guide to help the public prevent obesity and related chronic diseases. Their research, which involved more than a decade of conceptualization, testing, and political clearances, led to the pyramid-shaped food guide finally released in 1992. ▶

The design of the pyramid indicated that some foods should be eaten in greater amounts than others—a red flag to producers of meat and other foods in the "use sparingly" sectors. Meat industry lobbying induced the USDA to reexamine the research basis of the pyramid design and delay its release for a year. Nutritionists also had some concerns. Because portion sizes had expanded so much in the 1980s, they worried that advice to eat 6 to 11 servings of grain foods would promote obesity. Nevertheless, the pyramid proved useful and adaptable, was widely recognized, and survived until the more industry-friendly administration of George W. Bush.

In 2005, the Bush-era USDA released a new version of the pyramid cleansed of its "eat less" messages. Instead, it emphasized the less controversial "move more." ▶

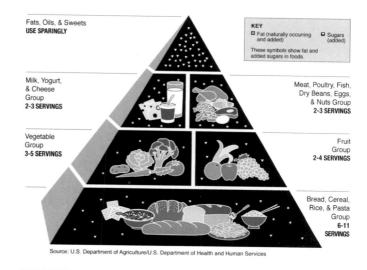

Fats, Oils, & Sweets
USE SPARINGLY

KEY
☐ Fat (naturally occurring and added)   ☐ Sugars (added)
These symbols show fat and added sugars in foods.

Milk, Yogurt, & Cheese Group
2-3 SERVINGS

Meat, Poultry, Fish, Dry Beans, Eggs, & Nuts Group
2-3 SERVINGS

Vegetable Group
3-5 SERVINGS

Fruit Group
2-4 SERVINGS

Bread, Cereal, Rice, & Pasta Group
6-11 SERVINGS

Source: U.S. Department of Agriculture/U.S. Department of Health and Human Services

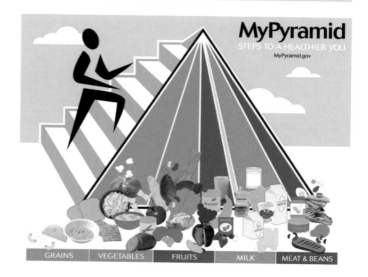

MyPyramid
STEPS TO A HEALTHIER YOU
MyPyramid.gov

GRAINS   VEGETABLES   FRUITS   MILK   MEAT & BEANS

To understand what the design meant, you had to use a computer to go online and discover that each of the rainbow stripes represented a distinct food group. Why would the USDA produce something so difficult to understand? Years of food industry lobbying had convinced USDA officials that nutritional judgments were controversial and good for neither business nor the USDA's mission to promote American agricultural products.

Many people found the new design confusing, not least because it seemed far removed from the reality of everyday eating habits. ▶ ▶

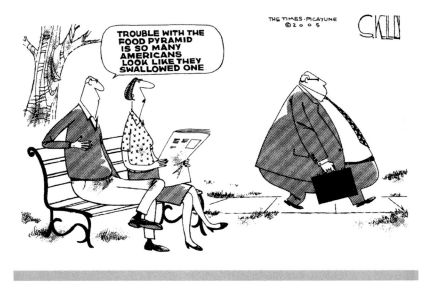

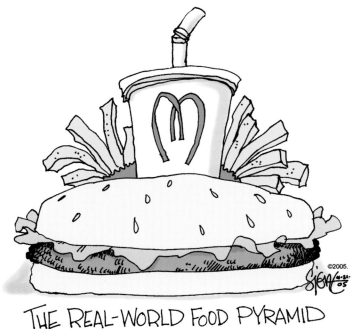

THE REAL-WORLD FOOD PYRAMID

THE OBAMA ADMINISTRATION'S INNOVATION: MYPLATE

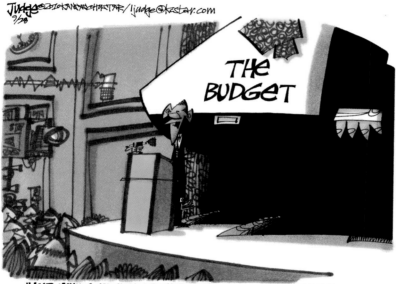

"AND WHILE MICHELLE DEALS WITH CHILDHOOD OBESITY..."

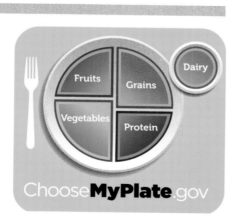

THE ELECTION OF President Barack Obama in 2008 introduced a fresh approach to food politics. Although the president was necessarily preoccupied with the need to improve the economy, reduce unemployment, and deal with the conflicts in Iraq and Afghanistan—at the same time under pressure to reduce government spending—First Lady Michelle Obama chose to use her position to try to reverse childhood obesity. ◄

A new food guide would help. In June 2011, the USDA introduced the Obama-era food icon: ChooseMyPlate. ◄

The plate is a sharp departure from previous food icons. It gives much greater prominence to foods from plant rather than animal sources. MyPlate pushes dairy foods

What Are We Supposed to Eat? **55**

off to the side and calls for vegetables, fruits, and grains on three-quarters of its space. Even so, its design can still confuse, as it allows considerable leeway in interpretation. People can pile whatever foods they like on plates of any size. Snacks and fast food do not require plates. ▼

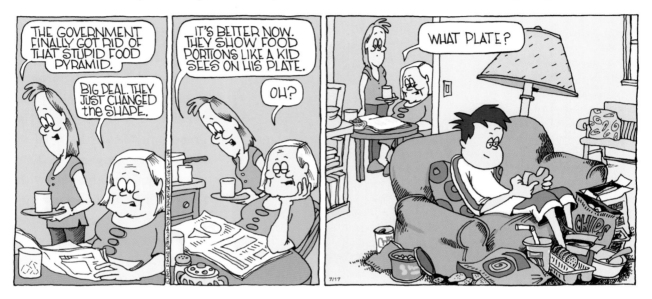

Dietary advice can always seem confusing, not least because it is impossible to capture the complexities of foods, diets, and body weight in one design or simple message. Much of the criticism of food icons is aimed at their design or ambiguous messages. In one sense, the confusion is ironic. The principal recommendations for preventing obesity and chronic disease were first issued in the 1950s and have not changed since: Eat more vegetables and other plant foods ("eat better"), balance calorie intake with physical activity ("move more"), and go easy on junk foods ("eat less"). If the constancy of dietary advice is not well understood, it is surely because advice to eat less of certain foods can affect their sales. Eating less, as I endlessly repeat, is bad for business. But another reason for public confusion stems from the difficulties involved in the design, conduct, and interpretation of nutrition research.

A PROBLEM: NUTRITION RESEARCH IS HARD TO DO

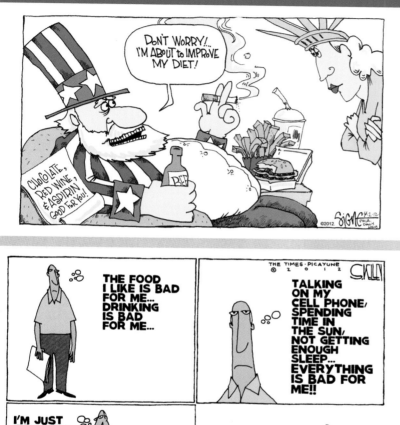

HUMANS MAKE TERRIBLE experimental animals. We vary in genetics, lifestyle, culture, and environment. We eat widely varying diets. And we are unable or unwilling to report what we eat or do with much accuracy. That is why researchers prefer to study animals or, if they must study human diets, investigate one nutrient or food at a time. The press finds the results of single-item research much more interesting to talk about than yawn-inducing advice to eat more vegetables. Everyone loves studies that contradict previous research, find harmful effects from eating favorite foods, show benefits from foods that are supposed to be bad for you, or emphasize the impossibility of ever doing anything right. ◄ ◄

Meat is particularly susceptible to cartoonists' commentary. Beef is high in saturated fat and cholesterol, and frequent consumption of beef is correlated with higher rates of chronic diseases. But is beef itself the problem, or is it merely a marker for generally unhealthful patterns of diet and health? Research studies cannot easily distinguish between the two possibilities. ▶ ▶

To distinguish the effects of one nutrient or one food from the effects of everything else people eat or do is not easy. Foods contain many nutrients, additives, and contaminants, any one of which might affect health. Diets vary from day to day. Typically, studies show small differences between groups consuming one diet or another—differences that show up only through the use of statistical tests. Human nutrition research requires

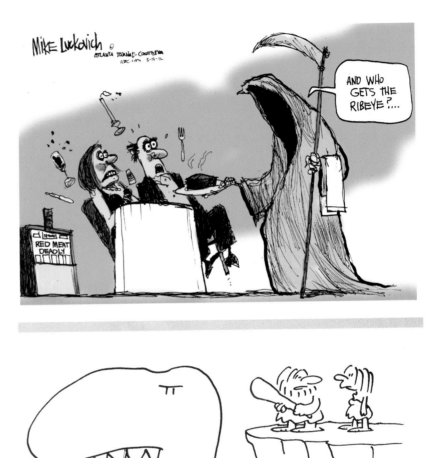

"Didn't I read somewhere that too much red meat isn't good for you?"

even more than the usual level of critical thinking in order to interpret the meaning of study results. But not everyone is careful to think critically about such things. Interpretation, as I keep saying, is invariably in the eye of the interpreter.

ANOTHER PROBLEM: DIETARY ADVICE IS HARD TO FOLLOW

IF DIETARY ADVICE seems complicated, it's also because following it can pose challenges. Most people pay little attention to dietary advice. Americans eat fewer vegetables, fruits, and whole grains than recommended, but far more junk foods. The leading sources of calories in American diets are "grain-based desserts," meaning such things as cupcakes, cookies, doughnuts, pies, and pastries. Bread, chicken products, soft drinks, pizza, and alcoholic beverages are also leading calorie sources.

Any number of studies and surveys document why people cannot easily eat healthfully.

- They may not understand the advice. ▼ ▶

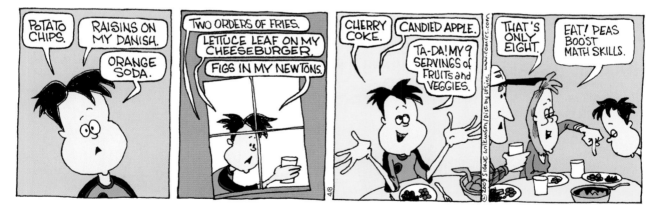

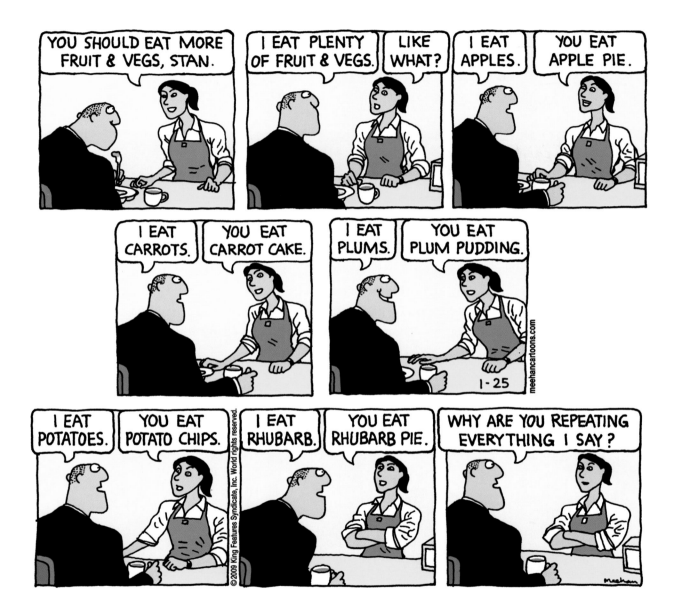

- They may not want to follow the advice. ▼ ▼

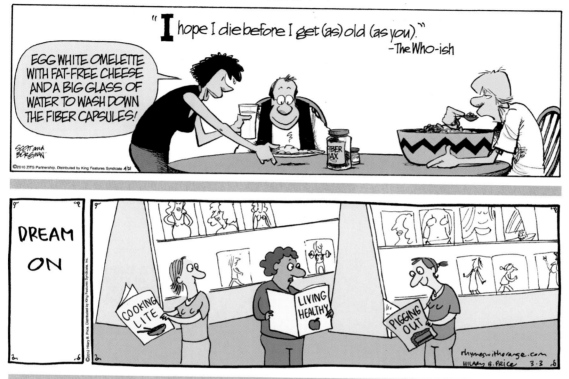

- They may want to follow the advice but find it inconvenient. ▼

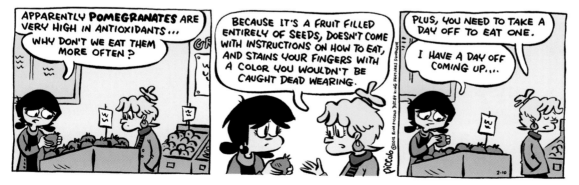

- They may be in denial about the need to eat healthfully. ▼ ▼

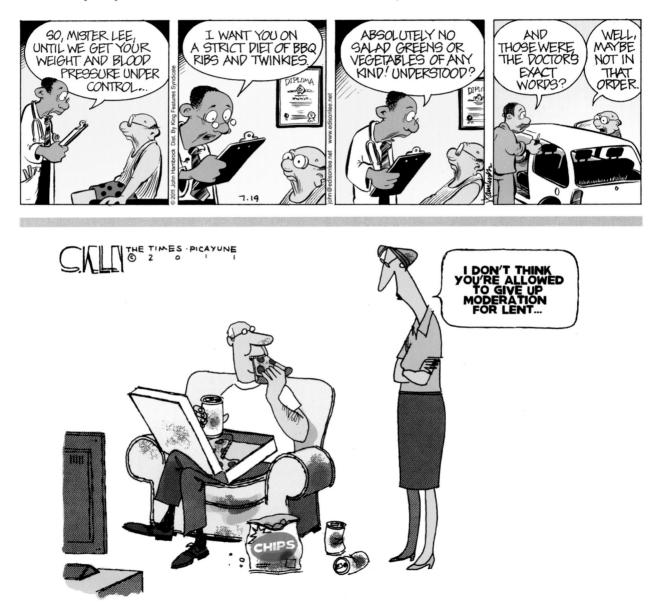

• They may feel they are being coerced into eating healthfully. ▼ ▼ ▼

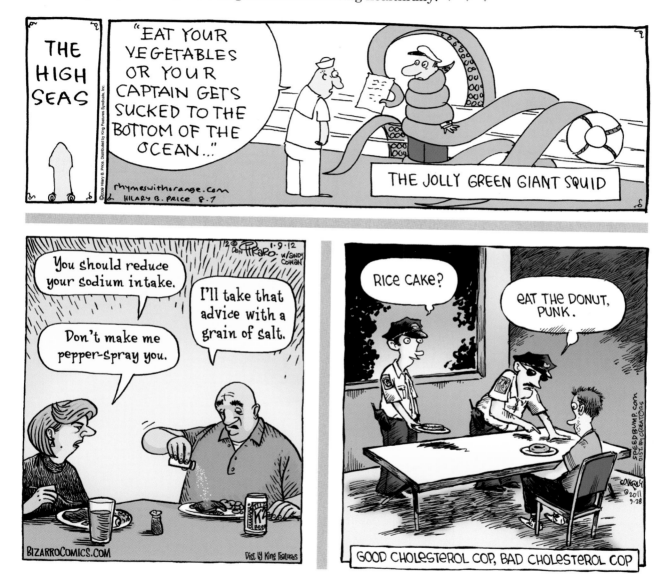

- They may want to eat more healthfully but can't afford to. ▼

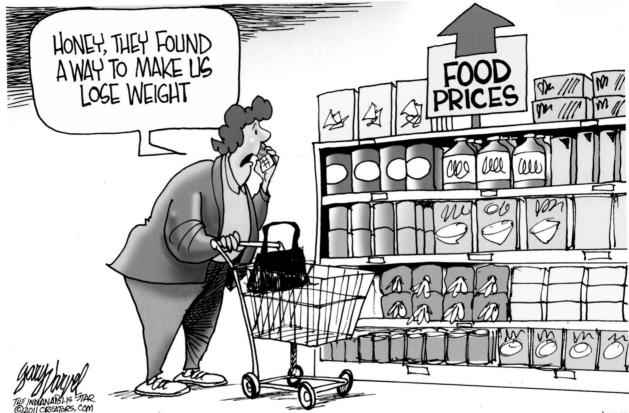

If fruits and vegetables appear more expensive than junk foods, it is because they are. Although USDA economists argue about the meaning of such figures, the Consumer Price Index indicates an increase of about 40 percent in the relative price of fruits and vegetables since the early 1980s, but a decrease in the indexed price of desserts, snack foods, and sodas by 20 to 30 percent. Higher prices discourage people from buying healthier foods. Prices are set by supply and demand, but also by agricultural policies that favor production of corn, soybeans, and other commodities used to feed farm animals and dairy cattle. ▼

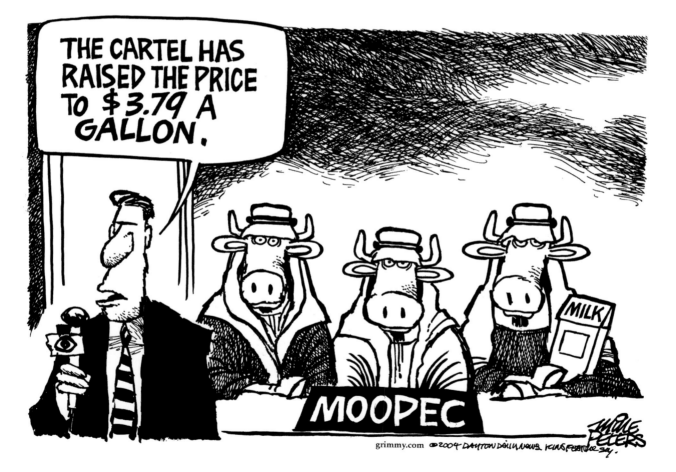

DOES IT MATTER WHEN WE EAT?

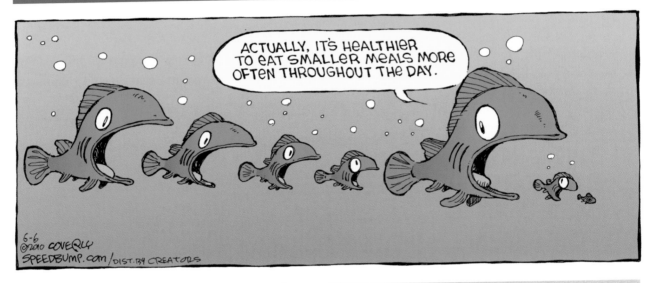

DIETARY GUIDELINES AND food guides have plenty to say about how much and what to eat, but little about how to space out meals. Dietary patterns differ so greatly among individuals that researchers have been unable to show that one or another pattern is better for health, weight, or longevity. ▲

Most nutritionists agree that breakfast is the most important meal of the day, but I am not one of them, at least when it comes to adults. I don't usually feel hungry until quite late in the morning. But research—much of it paid for by cereal companies—consistently reports that people who eat breakfast,

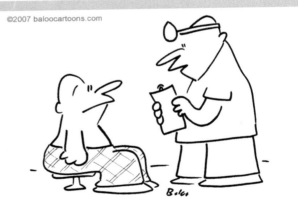

"You have a serious vitamin deficiency — Eat as much breakfast cereal as you can."

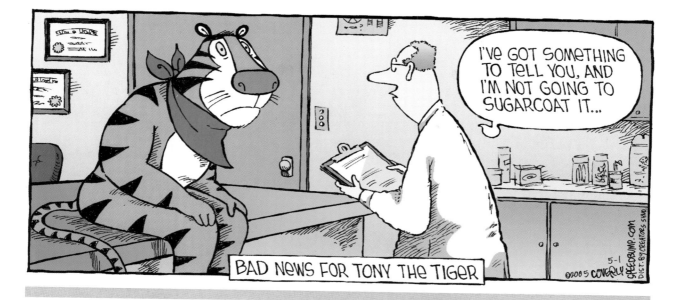

BAD NEWS FOR TONY THE TIGER

particularly vitamin-fortified breakfast cereals, are healthier than those who do not. ◄

Adults who don't like breakfast cereals, or who don't like breakfast at all, may object to being forced to eat foods they don't like. But it looks to me as if the makers of commercial breakfast cereals are those most likely to be harmed if adults don't eat their products. ▲

Children are another matter. Their digestive systems are smaller, they can't eat as much at any one time, and they do better and learn better in school when they eat something in the morning. What they are given for breakfast and, for that matter, at any time of day, is the topic of the next chapter. ▶

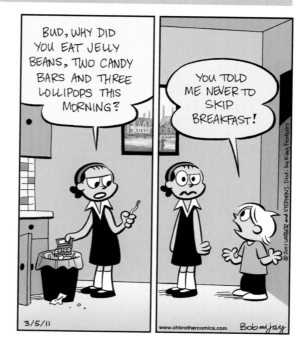

5 What about Feeding Kids?

THE PERSONAL RESPONSIBILITY ARGUMENT doesn't work for children. Most kids cannot choose their diets unless parents let them. You might never know it from the ways food companies market to kids and from the response to that marketing, but children are supposed to eat the same foods their parents eat. Dietary recommendations apply to everyone over the age of two. ▶ ▶

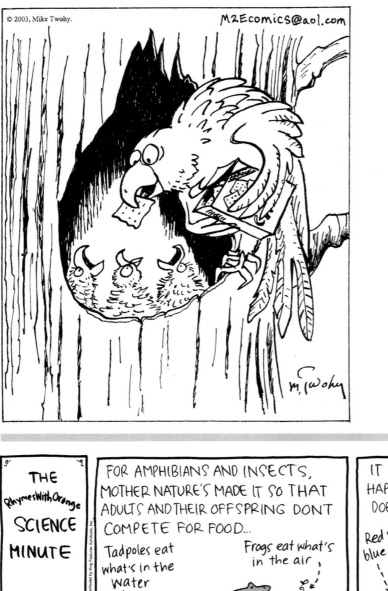

Once children are past infancy and can chew and swallow foods without choking, you can give them the same healthy foods that everyone else in the family is eating—just in smaller portions and with a few minor modifications: Leave out the salt and sugars, cut the foods into small pieces, and make sure the foods are well moistened so that small children don't choke on them. ▶

In an ideal world, parents eat healthy diets and kids happily eat whatever is served at home. But we do not live in an ideal world. Although children do not need soft drinks, juice drinks, desserts, candy, sweetened

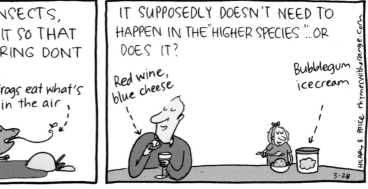

THE RhymesWithOrange SCIENCE MINUTE

FOR AMPHIBIANS AND INSECTS, MOTHER NATURE'S MADE IT SO THAT ADULTS AND THEIR OFFSPRING DON'T COMPETE FOR FOOD...

Tadpoles eat what's in the water

Frogs eat what's in the air

IT SUPPOSEDLY DOESN'T NEED TO HAPPEN IN THE "HIGHER SPECIES"...OR DOES IT?

Red wine, blue cheese

Bubblegum icecream

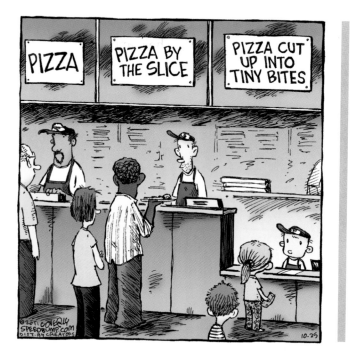

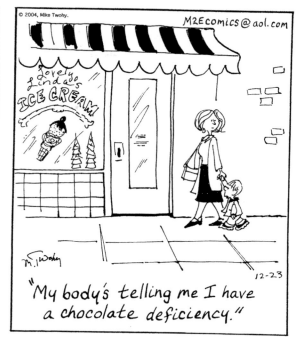

"My body's telling me I have a chocolate deficiency."

cereals, or fast food, they naturally like such foods. ▼

  Kids especially love candy and other sweet foods, and look for any excuse to eat them. ▲

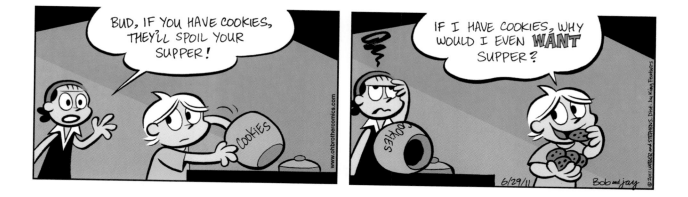

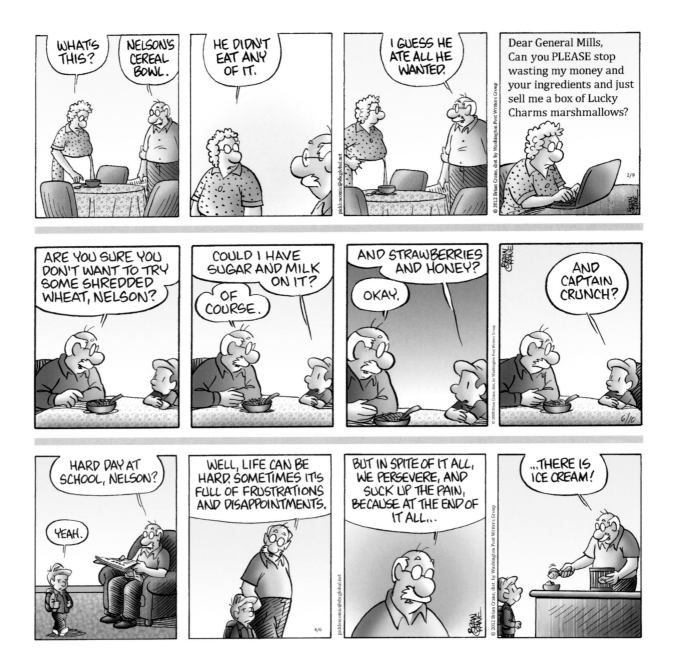

Food is a way to express love. Adults—particularly doting grandparents—enjoy indulging kids in what they most like to eat. ◄ ◄ ◄

In trying to make sure that kids eat healthfully, parents must face the facts: Some kids do not intuitively like eating healthfully. ▶

Researchers who study children's food preferences say that parents must expose their children to unfamiliar vegetables as many as 30 times before the kids will start accepting them. But this takes a degree of patience beyond that of all but the most diligent parents. ▼

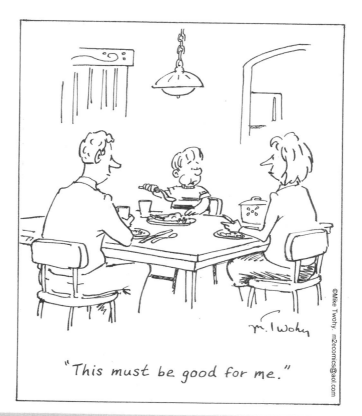

"This must be good for me."

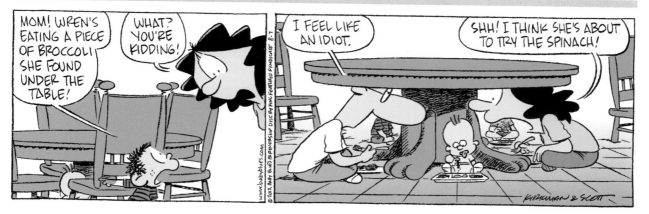

Instead, parents resort to threats, bribes, and seemingly endless negotiation to convince kids that they must eat what's good for them. ▼ ▼ ▼

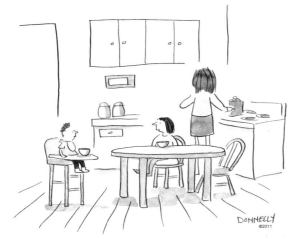

"You better eat that. People are starving in reality shows."

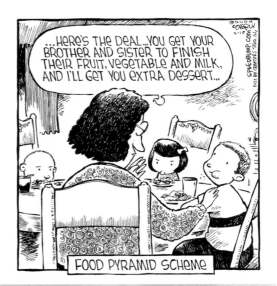

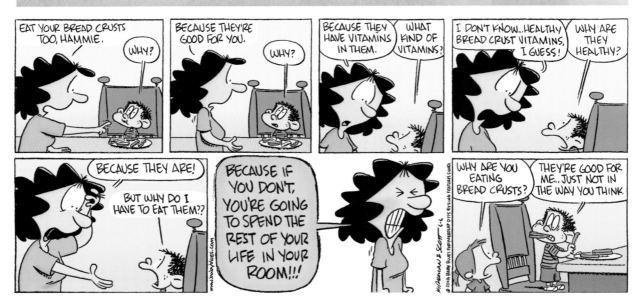

Parents who feel they have run out of options resort to "because I said so." ▼ ▼

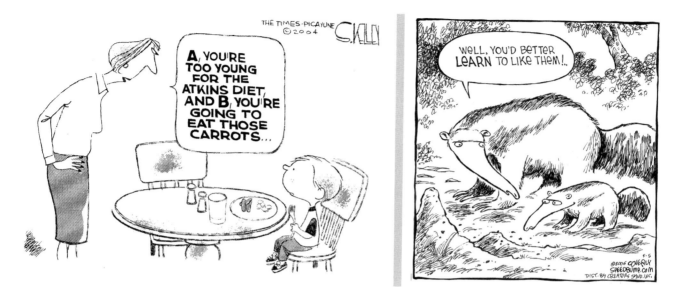

THE PROBLEM: MARKETING FOOD TO KIDS

IT IS ANYTHING but coincidental that kids prefer the very foods that are made and marketed to appeal to them. The amount of money that food advertisers spend to advertise directly to children can only be estimated, but it runs well into the billions. Any nationally advertised kids' food brand is backed by a budget of millions of dollars a year. For example, in 2011, Kellogg spent $51 million to advertise Pop-Tarts and $13.1 million to advertise Froot-Loops—just in the United States. McDonald's US advertising spending was $963 million that year. Do children naturally prefer junk food? Or do they like it because they are endlessly told that they should? Taste is critical, but research shows that children presented identical foods with and without advertised brand names greatly prefer the advertised products.

Food and beverage companies spend fortunes marketing their products to young children. ▼

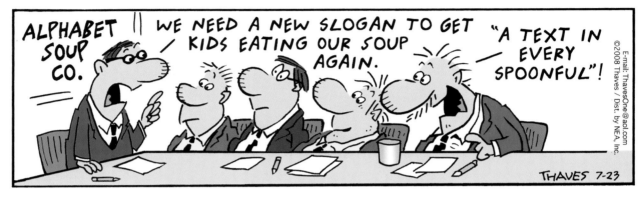

Even the most health-conscious parents I know—those who say they never let their kids watch TV, never take them to fast-food places, and never bring kids' cereals into the house—are astonished when their children ask for food products by name or plead to go to McDonald's. Marketing to children is so much a part of our culture that most of us do not even notice it. We are not *supposed* to. If the marketing is truly effective, we will not notice it. But kids do. They are particularly susceptible to marketing foods with toys. ▼ ▶

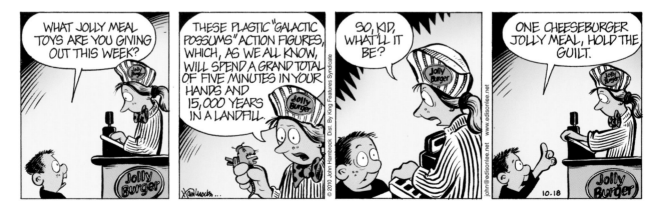

Why would marketers bother to spend so much time and money on kids, who have little money of their own? I can think of three reasons. The first is to encourage brand loyalty. The second is to get kids to pester their parents to buy the products. But the third reason is the most insidious. It's to get kids to believe that they are supposed to eat "kids' food," not the adult food served at home. It's to get them to believe that they know more about what they are supposed to eat than their parents do. Food marketing shifts the responsibility for deciding what children should eat from parents to the children themselves. As a result, meals become battlegrounds.

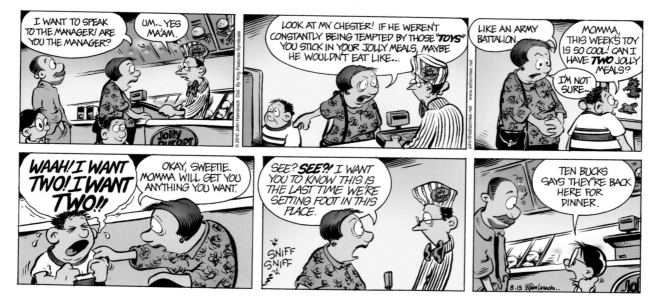

THE RESULT: CHILDHOOD OBESITY

NONE OF THIS would matter so much if kids remained healthy regardless of what they ate. But American children are gaining weight, and rapidly. More than one-third of American children and adolescents are overweight or obese, up from under 10 percent in 1980. Obesity is just as bad for the health and fitness of children as it is for adults. ▶

The reasons why kids are gaining weight are similar to those that explain adult obesity. The most obvious is eating too much of the wrong kinds of food. ▶

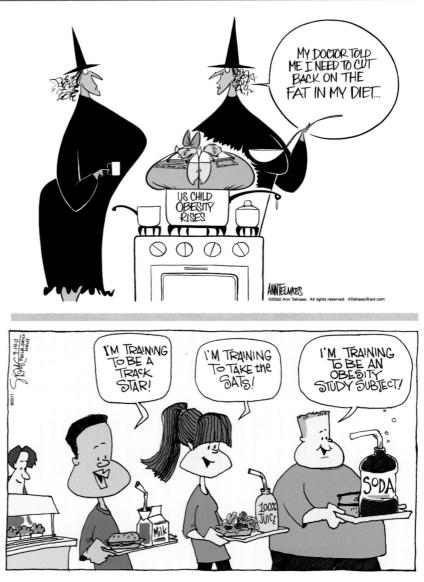

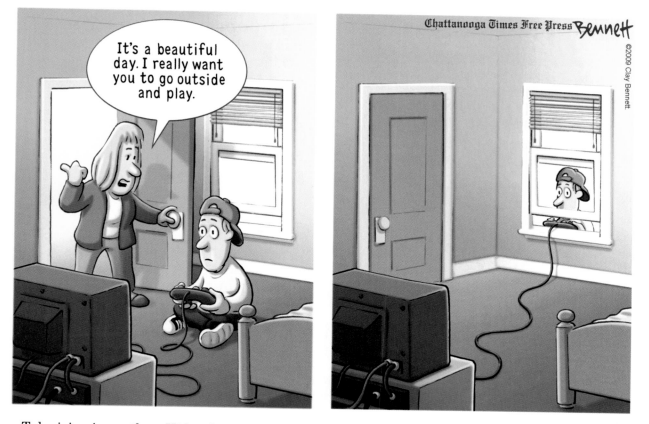

Television is another. Kids who watch a lot of TV are sedentary, deluged with commercials for junk foods and sodas, and snacking on what they see advertised. Pediatricians advise parents who are concerned about their kids' weight to keep media time to a minimum: Remove the TV from bedrooms, monitor TV watching and gaming, and mostly keep it turned off. ▲

But the effects of food marketing on kids' weight extend beyond advertising. Large food companies market their products in more subtle ways through "social responsibility" missions. They support research studies that demonstrate that the products do not affect body weight (independent studies tend to come to different conclusions). They also make large donations to community, sports, and

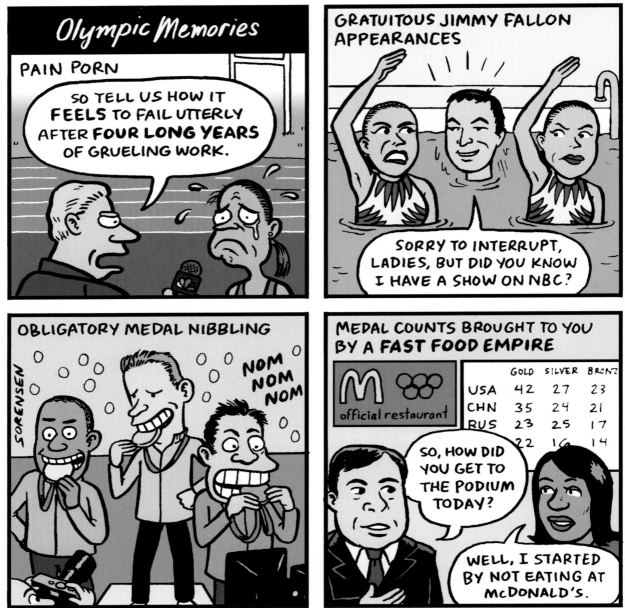

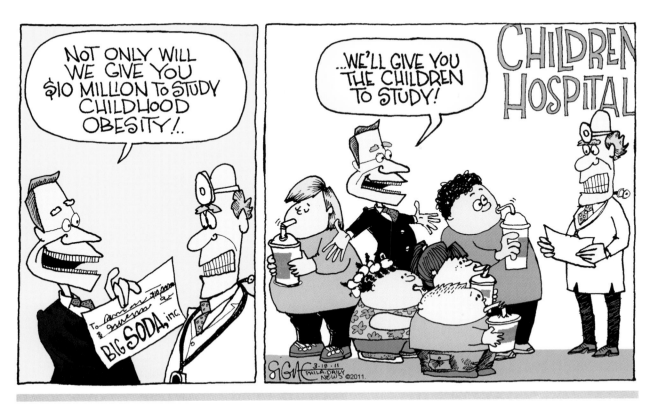

health organizations, children's hospitals among them. ◀ ▲

Perhaps you believe that it is unfair to attribute obesity to the effects of food industry marketing when the real problem is overly permissive parenting. ▶

Rather than wanting to see some limits set on food industry marketing, you might prefer government actions that focus on educating parents to do a

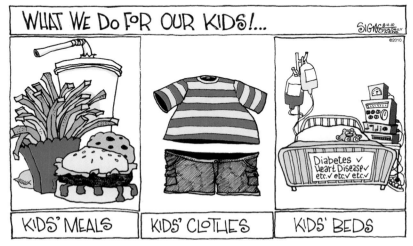

better job of managing what their kids eat. ▶

I agree that the job of parents is to set limits, but consider the enormity of what they are up against: an entire industry devoted to undermining their authority on food issues. Marketing to children does more than make kids want branded products. It subverts parental authority over food decisions. For this reason alone, marketing to children should be curtailed. And schools are a good place to start.

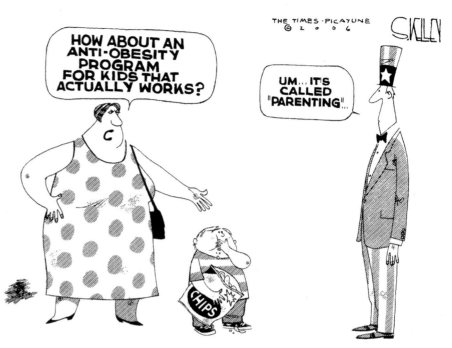

CAN SCHOOL FOOD BE FIXED?

SCHOOL MEALS HAVE long been the subject of scorn and not-so-fond memories of mystery meat. ▼

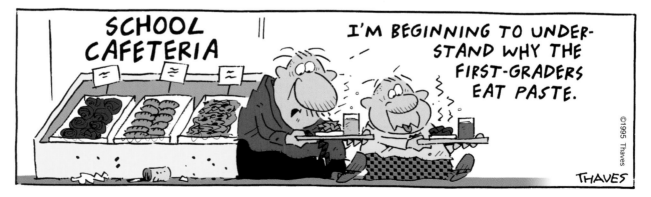

School meals provide a large portion of what many kids eat during the day. Whether schools want to or not, they set an example of what kids are supposed to eat. If schools serve poor quality food, and permit and encourage sales of sodas and snacks, they convey the idea that such foods are what kids are expected to eat every day.

Because school food service is supposed to pay for itself, schools have little choice but to buy what they serve at the lowest possible price. The USDA supports school meal programs so that low-income children can eat breakfast and lunch in school. It buys foods in bulk and provides them to schools at low cost. Cheap hamburger meat intended for school meals raises particular concerns about its origin and safety. ▼

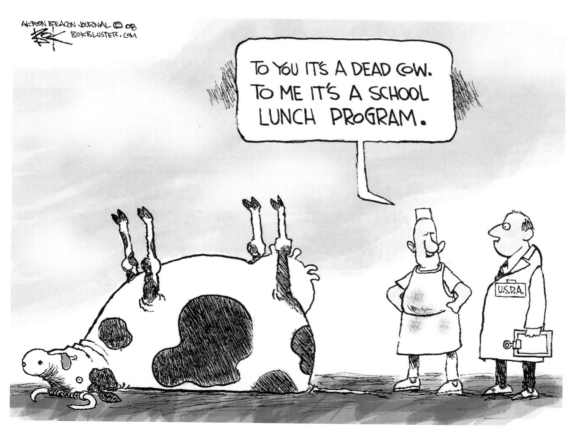

In 2012, concerned parents petitioned the USDA to stop adding a cheap "lean, finely textured beef" filler ingredient, more pejoratively known as "pink slime," to school hamburger. They particularly objected to the use of ammonia to kill pathogens in the meat trimmings used to produce this ingredient in their children's lunches. ▼

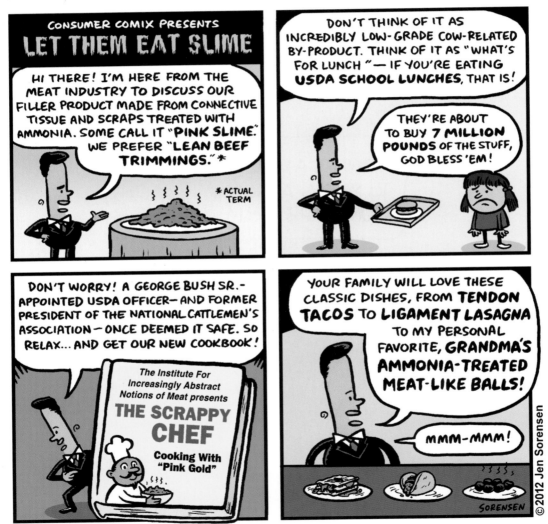

The USDA is committed to promoting healthful eating patterns and it provides guidelines for what children should eat on a regular basis. But serving healthy meals in schools can be challenging. If the foods don't taste good, the kids won't eat them.

School food service personnel may find it difficult to encourage kids to eat healthfully in schools where testing dominates the school day. ◣

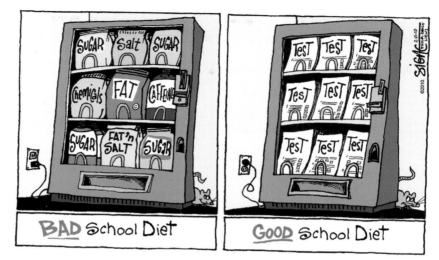

And sometimes schools transitioning to healthier meals find it necessary to train food service staff in the new approaches. ▼

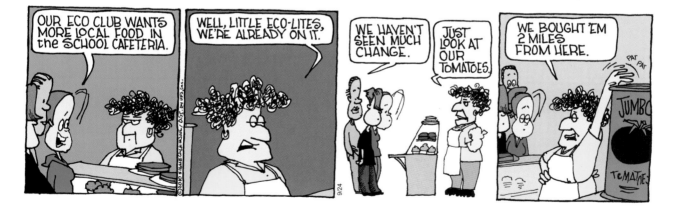

THE POLITICS OF FEEDING KIDS

YOU MIGHT NOT view school food as political, but providing nutritious breakfasts and lunches to schoolkids is the job of a large industry eager to stay in business and increase profits. In 2011, the USDA school breakfast program served nearly 12 million children at a cost of nearly $3 billion, while the much larger school lunch program served nearly 32 million children at a cost of $11 billion. The $14 billion in taxpayer dollars spent on these programs that year permitted many children who might otherwise go hungry to eat during the school hours. Any company involved in providing food for school meals—or in stocking foods and drinks sold in vending machines—wants its share of that money. ▲▼

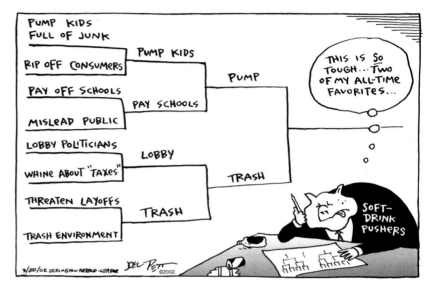

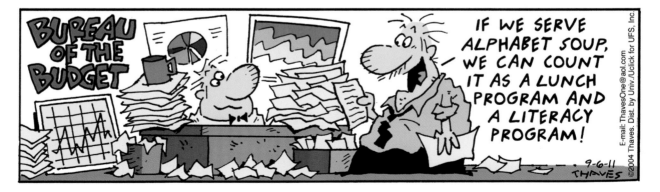

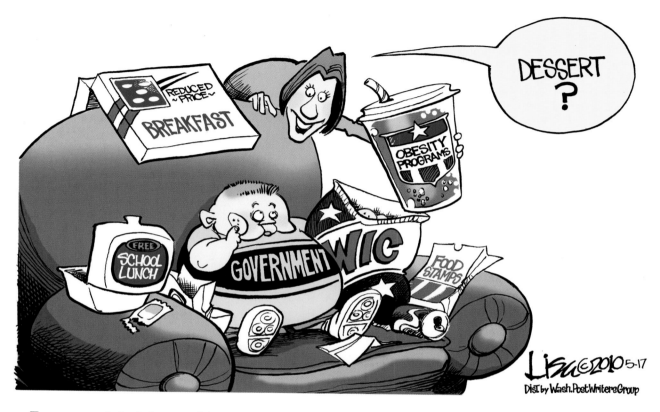

From my point of view, making sure that kids eat healthy meals is highly desirable public policy. Kids learn better when they aren't hungry. But people with different views of how society should work might consider school meals and other food assistance programs as prime examples of obesity-promoting government waste. ▲

The politics of school food is most evident in the controversy over setting nutrition standards for what is served. For all of the reasons why food marketers are in schools in the first place—a large, captive, impressionable audience with influence over parental purchases—schools are prime targets for obesity intervention. Schools across the country have transformed meal programs, but without a federal policy, these transformations had to be instituted school by school, with highly variable results.

In 2010, Congress passed the Healthy, Hunger-Free Kids Act, which authorized the USDA to establish nutrition standards for all food sold and served in schools, not only at breakfast and lunch, but also at any time during the school day. USDA's food-based proposals specified the number and size of servings of fruits, vegetables, meat, dairy, and grains. The agency also set nutrient-based standards for limits on saturated fat, trans fat, sodium, and calories. The limits troubled the food companies making products that did not meet the new standards. What to do? They went straight to Congress to weaken or overturn the new regulations. ▶ ▶

As I mentioned in the introduction, food industry lobbying succeeded in blocking USDA's proposed standard for the amount of tomato paste that could count as a vegetable serving. Previous USDA standards allowed ⅛ cup of tomato paste to

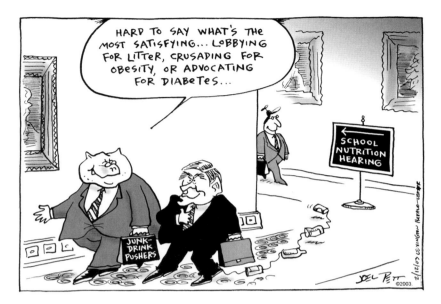

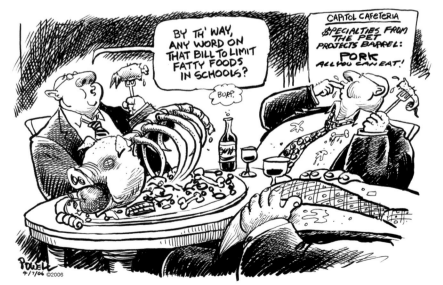

count, unlike any other fruit or vegetable; all others required at least ½ cup. Now the USDA was proposing to make tomato paste meet the same volume requirements as other fruits and vegetables. When the Senate chose to intervene, cartoonists went right to work. ▼ ▶

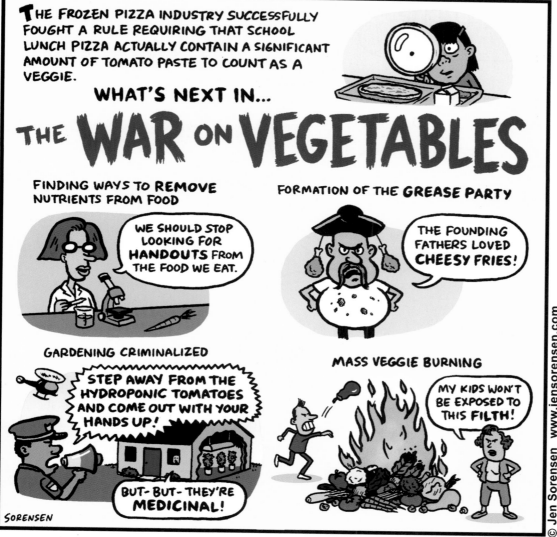

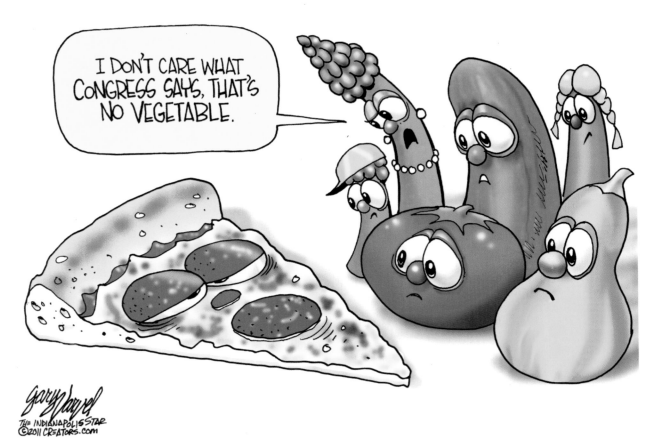

To promote public health, setting rigorous nutrition standards for school meals is the right thing to do. Children will be eating diets that meet their nutritional needs but do not encourage obesity. If you put the rights of individuals above all other considerations, however, you might view nutrition standards as unwarranted government interference in the private lives of citizens. ◤

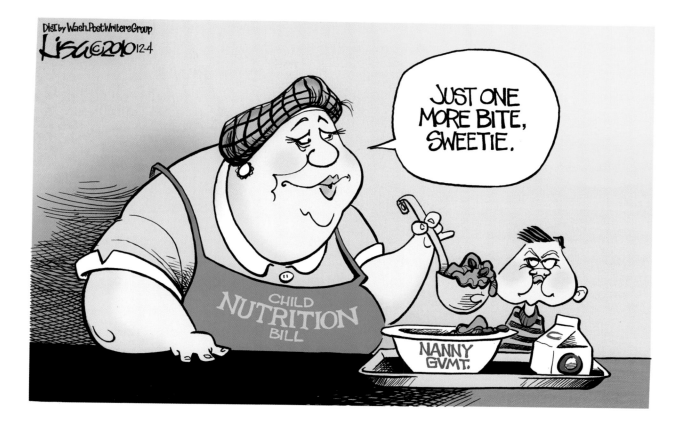

6 Food Issues: Who Decides?

AS WE HAVE SEEN, FOOD POLITICS AFFECTS a great many aspects of modern society. In my department at New York University, we explain Food Studies as a powerful lens through which to examine the most critical issues facing the world today. These include large, systemic problems—income inequality, racial and class prejudices, gender inequities, climate change, wars, and ethnic and religious conflicts—that are often decided by social and political forces far beyond the control of most individuals. But food issues also include smaller, more manageable matters over which individuals often can have substantial influence.

Among these less earth-shaking issues are day-to-day concerns about what to do about alcoholic beverages, whether to take dietary supplements, how to feed pets, what to do about food safety, and whether to eat foods that have been genetically modified or come from cloned animals. Cartoonists have much to say about such matters, often using them as ways to comment on the larger issues confronting society.

ALCOHOLIC BEVERAGES

ALCOHOLIC BEVERAGES HAVE been consumed throughout human history, but drinking too much of them poses dilemmas for individuals and for society. Drinking and binge drinking induce people to act irresponsibly and cause automobile and gun accidents, violence, and abuse. But advice about alcohol is complicated by observations that consuming it in moderation reduces the risk of coronary heart disease. ▼

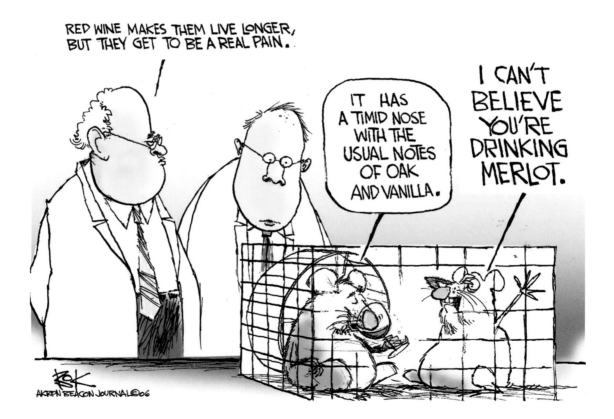

Only about half of Americans drink alcohol regularly. About 9 percent of men and 4 percent of women consume more than the recommended upper limit: two drinks a day for men and one for women. It is just these heavy drinkers, particularly those who binge, who are at higher risk for injuries, violence, liver cirrhosis, high blood pressure, stroke, diabetes, and, in women, breast cancer. Because of these risks, health authorities rarely advise anyone who does not drink to start. They cite other ways to reduce heart disease risk—eating healthfully, for example. ▶

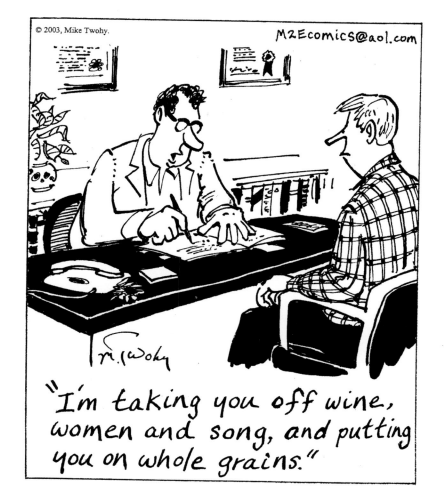

One further concern about alcohol has to do with its calories. Alcohol is almost as fattening as fat—7 calories per gram—and its calories can add up just like those from any other source. As with much else about diet, moderation is the best advice. ▶

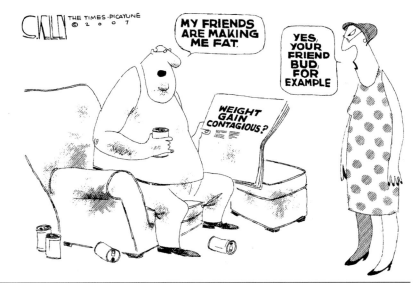

VITAMIN SUPPLEMENTS

AMERICANS BOUGHT MORE than $11 billion worth of vitamins in 2009, and these accounted for about one-third of all dietary supplement sales. Despite the lack of evidence that vitamin supplements make healthy people healthier, more than half of American adults take these products in the hope that they will make up for dietary deficiencies, compensate for poor diets, and guarantee health and longevity. ▶

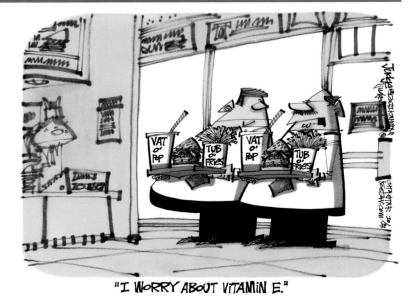

"I WORRY ABOUT VITAMIN E."

The supplement industry exploits fears of dietary inadequacy to try to convince the public that the products are essential and that it's easier to get nutrients from supplements than to bother about what's in the daily diet. Cartoonists have no trouble capturing the ironies of supplement marketing. ▶

For most people, vitamins are best obtained from foods, and supplements are rarely necessary. ▼

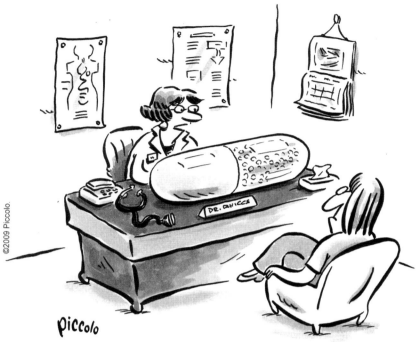

"With this all-in-one vitamin you won't need any other vitamin."

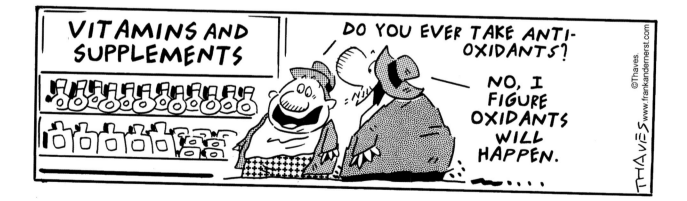

PET FOODS

THE CARE OF PETS is an enormous industry in the United States, one worth more than $50 billion a year. Americans own nearly 90 million cats and 80 million dogs, all of them needing to be housed, cared for, fed, and, in many households, pampered. Feeding constitutes a third or more of expenditures on pets. Hundreds of firms manufacture pet food products, but five companies control 80 percent of the market: Nestlé Purina (no relation), Mars, Hill's (Colgate-Palmolive), Iams (Procter & Gamble), and Del Monte.

Dogs will eat almost anything, but cats are carnivores and fussier. Before the invention of commercial pet food, cats ate mice, while dogs were fed table scraps or left to forage on human-food leftovers or garbage. Commercial pet foods made

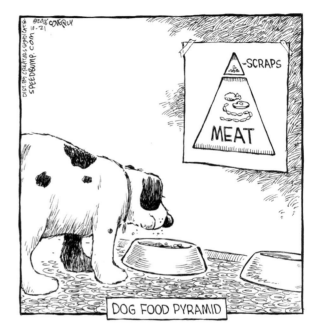

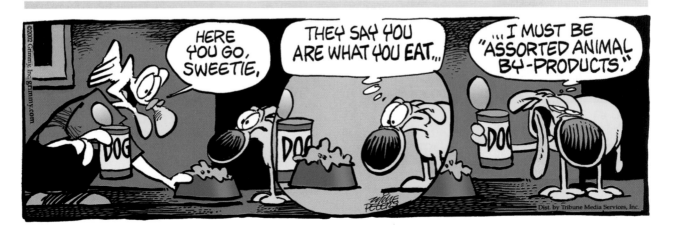

feeding cats and dogs easier for owners to manage. They also solved the problem of what to do with the nutritious by-products of human food production that would otherwise go to waste. By-products can provide all of the nutritional needs of dogs or cats in one convenient can, but their very name invokes disgust. By-products, after all, are the parts of food animals—the organs, fat, bone, and trim—that we choose not to eat. Whether revolting to us or not, commercial pet foods are specifically formulated to support the animals' nutrient needs, growth, and reproduction. ◀ ◀

With so many questionable ingredients included as by-products, it makes sense to ask whether it is safe to feed commercial products to pets. Occasionally, pet food companies have recalled products found to contain toxins or salmonella.

In 2007, manufacturers recalled nearly 100 brands of pet foods that contained melamine, an industrial chemical used to make plastic dinnerware. As I explained in *Pet Food Politics,* unscrupulous ingredient suppliers in China had used melamine as a replacement for expensive protein ingredients in pet food. Melamine is high in nitrogen and appears as protein in laboratory tests. Unlike protein, melamine has no nutritional value. Worse, melamine is degraded in the body to chemicals with which it can combine to form crystals that destroy kidney function. The tainted pet food caused the death of untold numbers of dogs and cats. I viewed this event as a classic case of failure in international food safety regulation. If this could happen to dogs and cats, the human food supply was also at risk. ▶

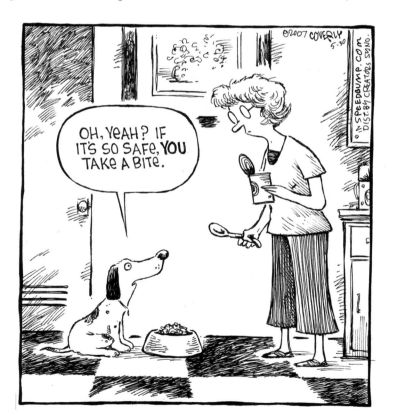

GENETICALLY MODIFIED FOODS

GENETICALLY MODIFIED ORGANISMS (GMOs) are inherent fodder for satire. To modify food crops, geneticists harvest genes from plants, bacteria, or viruses to transfer some desirable characteristic into the crops, such as corn or soybeans. The most commonly transferred characteristics are resistance to insects or to weed killers such as Roundup (glyphosate), but the biotechnology industry also promises genetically modified improvements in the nutritional quality of foods. ◥

These kinds of genetic manipulations evoke visions of Frankenstein monsters and mad scientists, as well as fears of corporate control of the food supply and collusion with government agencies to foist unwanted foods on a hapless public. ▶ ◥

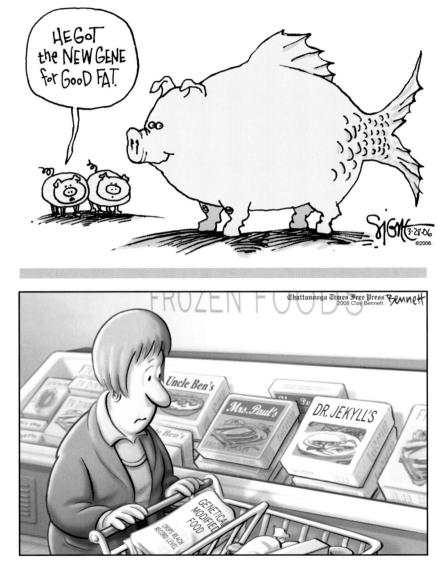

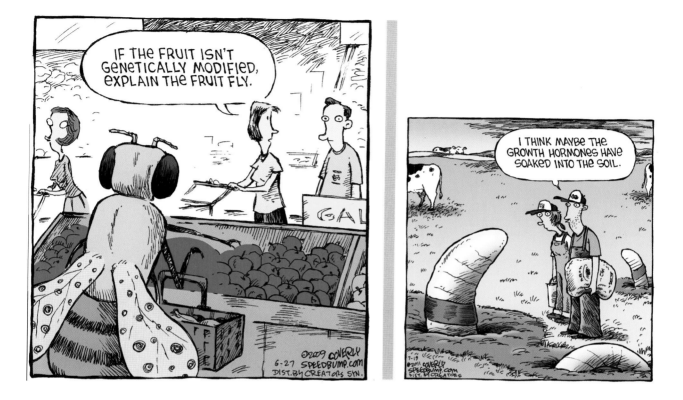

The science of GMOs is complicated and difficult to evaluate, even for people who have been trained in science as I was. Technology that is not well understood comes across to many people as especially bizarre or frightening. In the United States, Monsanto introduced a hormonal drug produced through genetic modification—recombinant bovine growth hormone (more formally, recombinant bovine somatotropin)—to induce cows to produce greater quantities of milk. This hormone elicited immediate controversy. Critics were concerned about what it might do to cows, to milk, and to people who drank milk from cows treated with the hormone. International trading partners objected and insisted that they would not accept imports of genetically modified food products. ▲

Food biotechnology companies argue that their technical innovations are essential for meeting the food needs of the world's burgeoning population, are safe, and produce substantial benefits for consumers as well as farmers. ▼

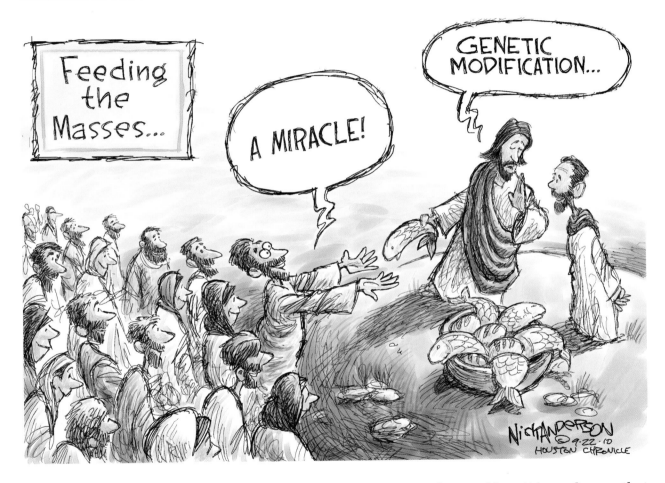

Whether these claims are true is debatable. Critics of the technology and how it is used argue that the main benefits of GMOs do not accrue to the public, but instead are created for the benefit of biotechnology corporations. As evidence, they note how aggressively the companies defend their patent

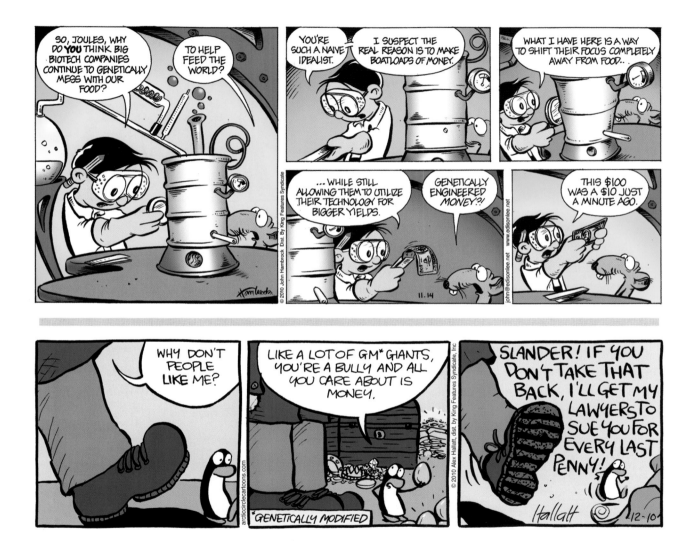

rights. Instead of focusing on the food needs of the developing world, food biotechnology companies engage almost exclusively in research on first-world agriculture: genetically modified corn, soybeans, and cotton bioengineered to resist weed killers made by those very same corporations. ▲ ▲

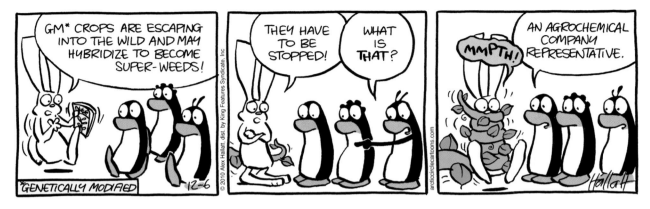

Critics also point out that the widespread use of glyphosate weed killers has caused natural selection for "superweeds" resistant to these herbicides. Roundup-resistant weeds have proliferated, and more pesticides than ever are needed to keep them under control. ▲

Whether the foods are safe is another matter of debate. Little evidence suggests that the foods cause demonstrable harm to human health, but the strangeness of the technology and uncertainties in the science can make people uncomfortable about eating GMOs. ▼

A large part of the discomfort, in my opinion, has to do with lack of transparency. When the FDA approved genetically modified foods for production and sale in the United States in 1994, the agency ruled that no special labeling was needed. The FDA's rationale: GMOs were no different from foods created through conventional genetic crosses. But without labeling, you have no idea whether you are

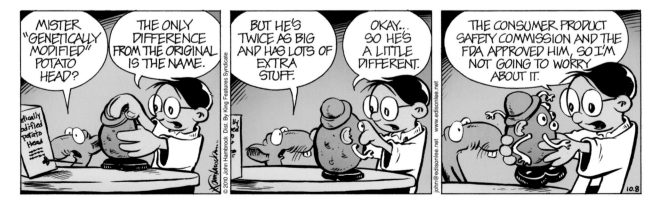

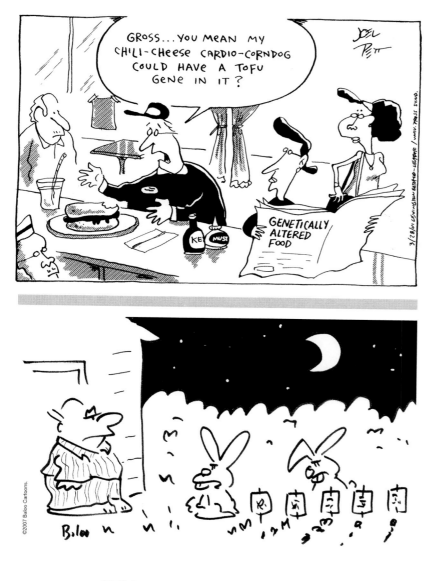

"This stuff isn't genetically engineered, is it?"

eating GMOs when you go out to a restaurant. ◀

Since 1994, the FDA has approved genetically modified foods such as ripening-delayed tomato and cantaloupe; herbicide-resistant soy, corn, canola, and sugar beets; insect-resistant corn, tomato, and potato; virus-resistant papaya and squash; and sterile radicchio.

In *Safe Food: The Politics of Food Safety,* I explain the clashing viewpoints about GMOs as expressions of differing value systems—those based mostly on science ("GMOs are safe; therefore, they are acceptable") as opposed to those that also include concerns about the cultural, religious, and political implications of the foods ("Even if GMOs are safe, they are not necessarily acceptable"). But one aspect of the GMO controversy is self-evident. In the United States at least, consumers do not have a choice. Genetically modified foods are not labeled. ◀

At the time of this writing, pressure was building to induce the FDA to authorize GMO labeling. The agency was still considering what to do about salmon genetically modified to grow faster, but appeared to be leaning toward approval. Many Americans might be more willing to accept such foods if they were labeled. That way, those who care about this issue would have a choice. ▼

As long as GMO foods remain unlabeled, they are likely to continue to elicit fear and distrust of not only the biotechnology industry, but also its federal regulators.

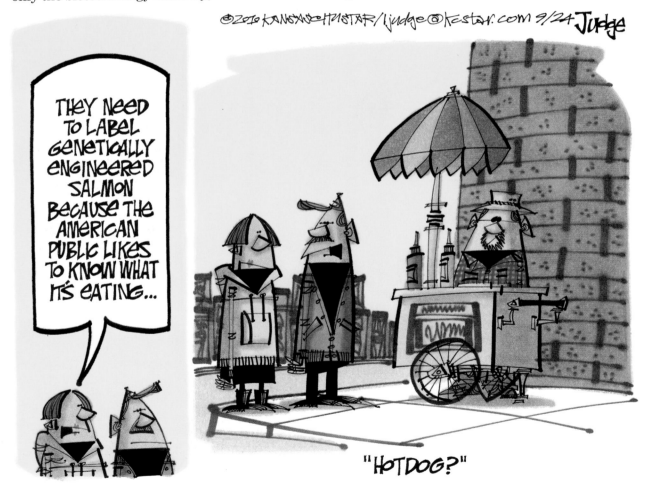

CLONED ANIMALS

IF THE IDEA of GMO foods seems strange, then eating meat from cloned animals seems even more so. ▶

Animal cloning began in 1996 with a sheep called Dolly, a laboratory creation from an egg from a female sheep. Scientists took the egg and removed its nucleus (the part containing the genes). They inserted a different nucleus into the egg, one taken from cells of the sheep they wanted to copy. They implanted the resulting embryo—Dolly—into the uterus of a surrogate sheep, who carried the lamb to term and delivered her in the usual manner. ▼

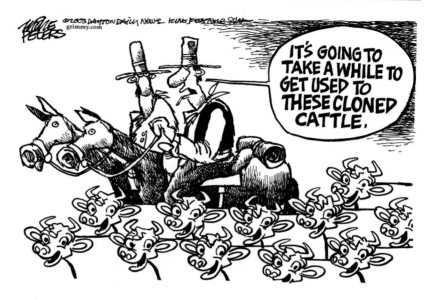

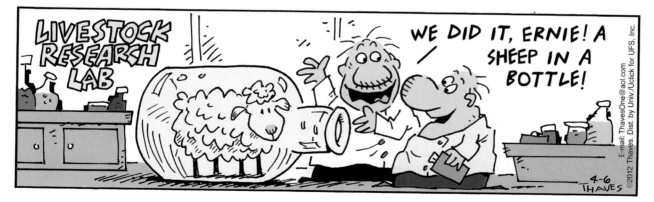

Cloning allows farmers to copy their best stock—animals that resist disease, produce the most milk, are most fertile, or have the best meat. ▼

Cloned animals are mostly used for breeding stock, but their offspring go into the food supply. To date, more than 20 kinds of animals have been cloned, but the ones most commonly used for food in the United States are cows, pigs, and goats. The FDA says these are safe for human consumption, "similar to identical twins, only born at different times. … A clone is not a mutant, nor is it a weaker version of the original animal."

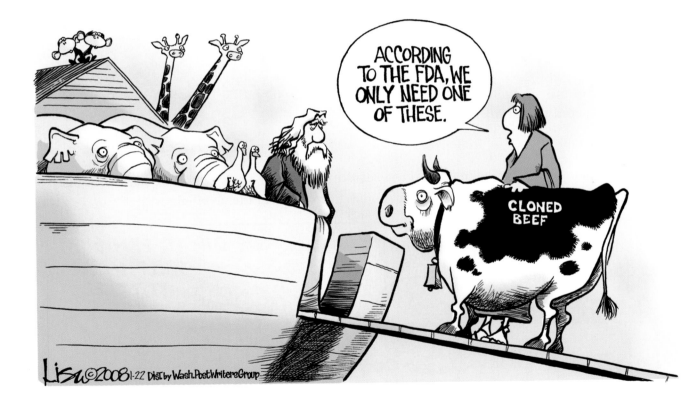

Are offspring from cloned animals in the food supply? Yes, they are. Would you be interested in knowing whether you are eating meat from a cloned animal? As with GMOs, the FDA says that because cloned animals are no different from any other food animal, their meat does not have to be labeled in any special way. But, at the same time, the FDA recommends that cloned species other than cows, pigs, and goats be kept out of the food supply due to lack of information about how people will respond to them. ▼

Without labeling, the public has no choice about consuming meat from cloned animals. For many people, the lack of choice is a principal rationale for buying organic foods and a major stimulant to the organic industry, as I discuss in Chapter 10.

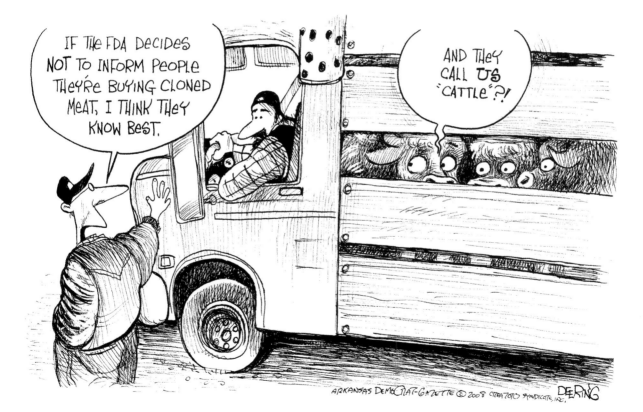

7

Food Safety: Who Is Responsible?

HOW COULD SOMETHING LIKE FOOD SAFETY BE political? Who would not want food to be safe? But consider what it takes to get food to the table. The American food system ranges from fields to kitchens and employs millions of people. Vegetables grow in soil, food animals excrete, and people carry diseases. Bacteria, viruses, and chemicals can easily contaminate foods and sicken anyone who eats them. Indeed, as Secretary of Health and Human Services Tommy Thompson famously said when he resigned from his post in 2004, "I, for the life of me, cannot understand why terrorists have not attacked our food supply because it is so easy to do." ▶

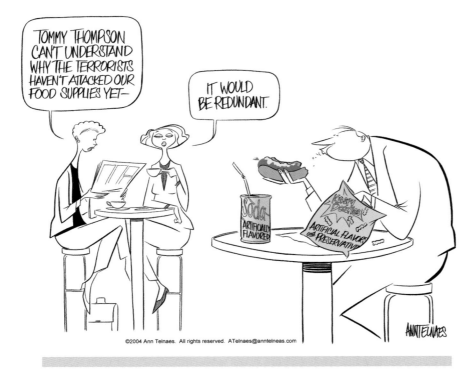

The vulnerability of the food supply can be explained in large part by weaknesses in the country's food safety system. In essence, food safety regulation is divided between two federal agencies: the USDA for meat and poultry, and the FDA for all other foods. ▼

For reasons of history, both agencies are funded through congressional agriculture appropriations committees, even though the FDA is a unit of Tommy Thompson's old health department. One result is that the FDA gets one-quarter of the funding for food safety even though it is responsible for three-fourths of the food supply.

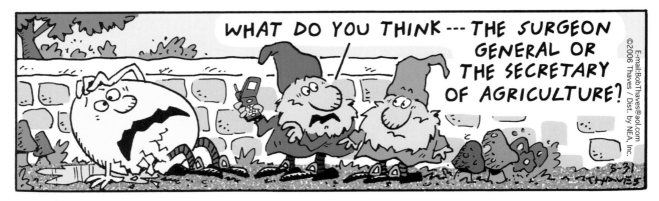

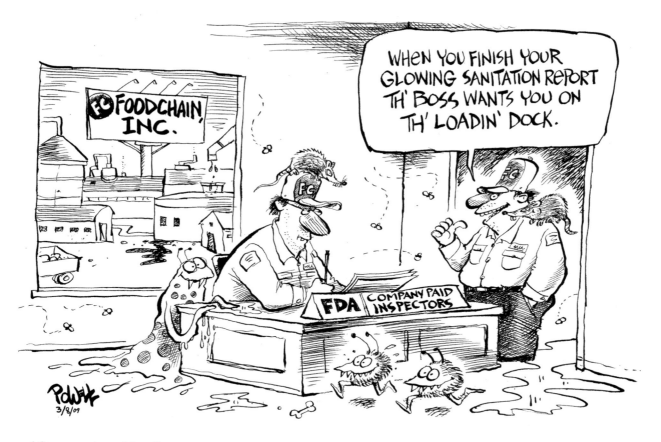

After a series of deadly outbreaks of foodborne illness, two of which I discuss below, Congress began working to strengthen food safety legislation and late in 2010 passed the FDA Food Safety Modernization Act. This act enabled the FDA to require and enforce prevention measures, inspect farms and production facilities, and recall contaminated foods. It also allowed the FDA to collect user fees from the companies being inspected, raising questions of conflict of interest. ▲

The FDA did not propose rules to implement this law for a full two years. What held them up? The food industry always prefers to manage food safety on a voluntary basis, but these particular rules got caught in 2012 election-year politics when reductions in government spending and regulation emerged as major points of contention.

PROBLEMS WITH FOOD safety regulation sprang to public attention in the early 2000s when one food after another became implicated in disease outbreaks. The CDC estimated that food-borne microbial illnesses affected 48,000 people a year and caused 128,000 hospitalizations and 3,000 deaths. Many of these were caused by toxic forms of common intestinal bacteria such as E. coli and salmonella, which soon became household words. ▶

These bacteria are fecal contaminants derived from farm animals. Meat production is inherently dirty, and contaminated meat has long been recognized as a cause of illness. ▶

But in recent years, vegetables such as spinach have been more frequently identified as sources of outbreaks. These leafy greens,

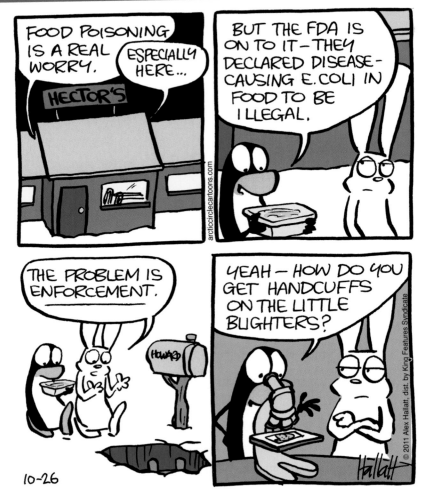

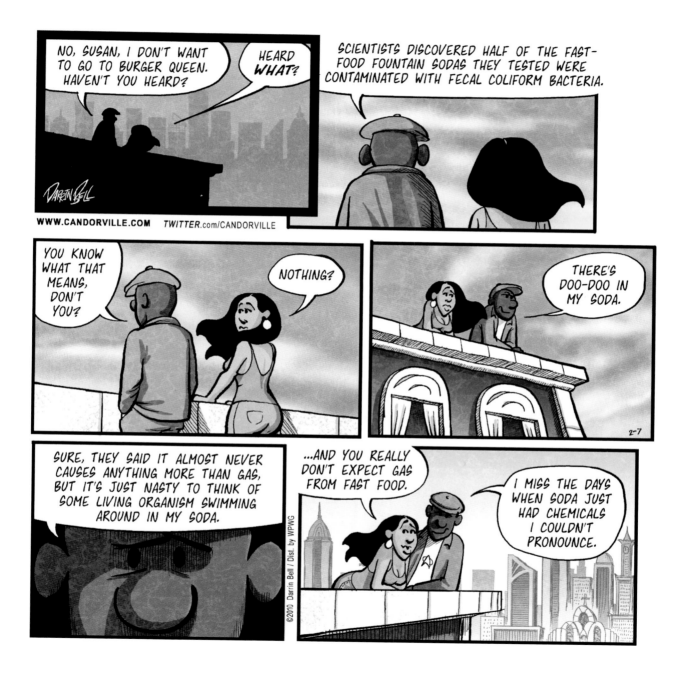

often eaten raw, must have come into contact with animal wastes—collateral damage from our increasingly industrialized and concentrated animal production and food distribution systems. ▶

The USDA's approach to food safety requires meat and poultry producers to follow preventive procedures, but also places considerable responsibility on individual households and consumers. Its education campaigns urge the public to follow basic food safety procedures: clean, separate, cook, chill. ▶

This is excellent advice. Everyone should adhere to basic food safety procedures at home. But shouldn't food be safe when it arrives in the home? And what about restaurants? They too should be required to adhere to food safety

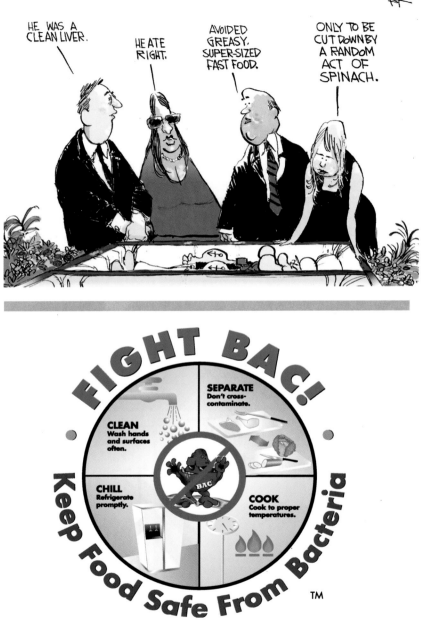

standards and take every possible precaution to protect customers from foodborne illness. ▶

Critics of government regulation argue that no legislation can protect citizens from dangerous microbes, not least because so much food is imported from countries with food safety systems even less effective than ours. The new food safety law gives the FDA greater authority to oversee imported foods. But Congress did not necessarily provide the FDA with additional funds to carry out its new responsibilities. ▼

With this background, let's take a look at two of the outbreaks that induced Congress to pass the Food Safety Modernization Act.

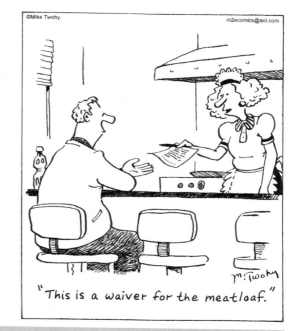

"This is a waiver for the meatloaf."

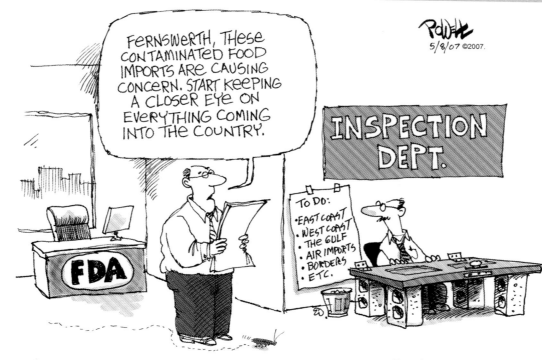

CONTAMINATED PEANUT BUTTER

You might not imagine that peanut butter could be a source of deadly bacteria, but peanuts are grown on soil and packed in factories that are not always as clean as one would wish. Late in 2008, the CDC investigated a large salmonella outbreak that affected nearly 500 people. Of these, nearly 80 percent recalled eating peanut butter before they got sick. ▼

The CDC traced the peanut butter to manufacture by the Peanut Corporation of America (PCA). It

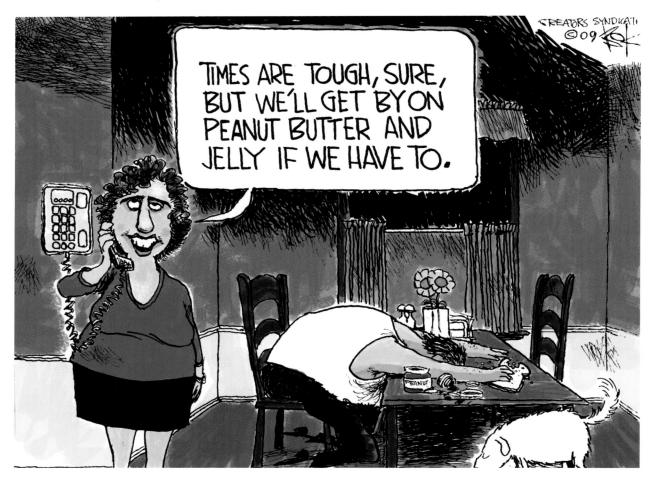

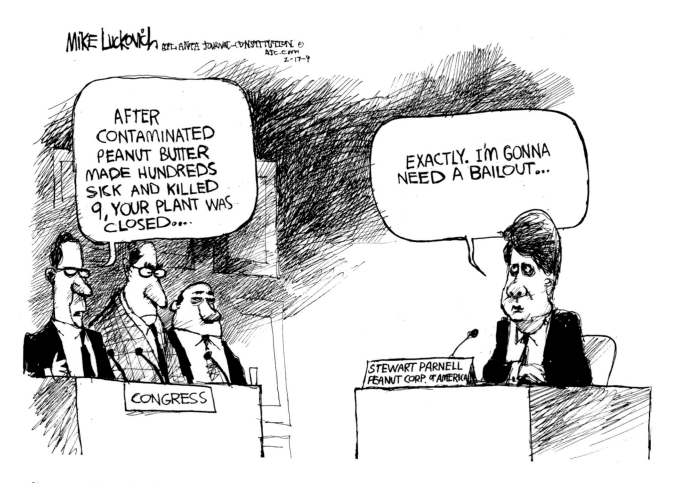

discovered that the PCA knew that tests for salmonella had come back positive, but the company had the samples retested until the results came back negative. Despite hazardous production standards, the company had passed inspections. Its president, Stewart Parnell, was called to explain his actions to Congress, but efforts to bring him to a grand jury were delayed or abandoned. As of mid-2013, he was awaiting trial. ▲

The PCA eventually recalled nearly 4,000 food products containing its peanut butter—crackers, frozen chicken, emergency disaster rations, and pet foods—and filed for bankruptcy protection. Although this incident induced Congress to agree to food safety legislation, it left consumers in a quandary about whether it was safe to buy peanut butter. ▶

CONTAMINATED EGGS

In 2010, a company in Iowa agreed to a "voluntary" recall of half a billion eggs linked to salmonella illness among nearly 2,000 people. After-the-fact investigations revealed a long history of safety violations and unsanitary conditions at the egg-producing facility, further emphasizing the need for stronger federal regulation of this and other safety matters. ▶

By 2013, the owner of the egg facility also had not been prosecuted, sending a message that when it comes to food safety matters, food producers have a good chance of getting away with whatever damage they cause.

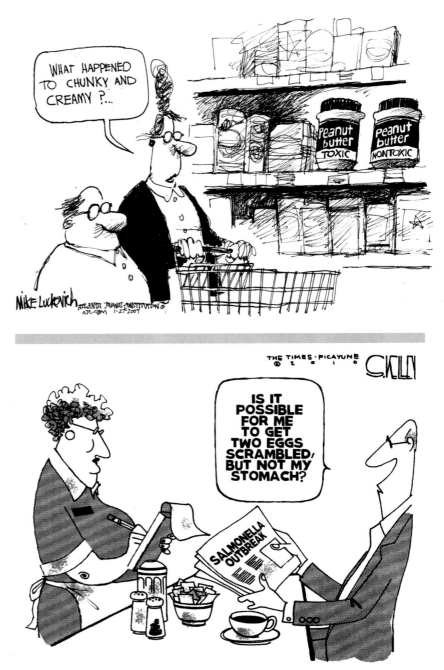

WHY NOT IRRADIATE?

SOME FOOD SAFETY experts say that the country cannot afford to wait for food safety regulation and must act now to protect people from microbial safety hazards. The answer, they say, is irradiation. This process involves bombarding foods with high-energy gamma rays, x-rays, or as is most common these days, electron beams. These kill bacteria with reasonable efficiency and do not make foods radioactive. But this kind of technological approach to food safety makes many people so uncomfortable that irradiation techniques are not widely used. ▶

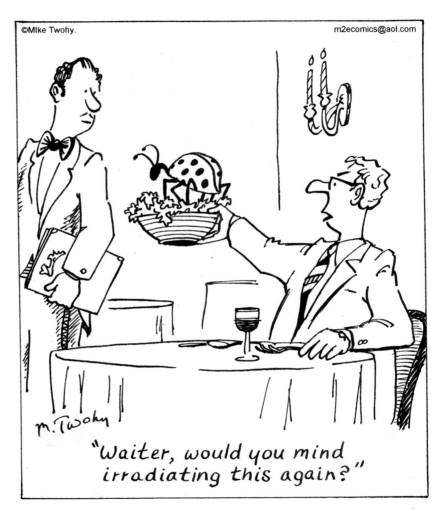

WHAT ABOUT CHEMICAL CONTAMINANTS?

MICROBIAL CONTAMINANTS MAY be the most serious cause of immediate foodborne illnesses, but people worry most about the long-term consequences of consuming agricultural pesticides and industrial chemicals. These cannot be seen, smelled, or tasted; cannot be under personal control; and are not monitored to an extent that might reassure the public. How they stack up against other food safety hazards is uncertain. ▼

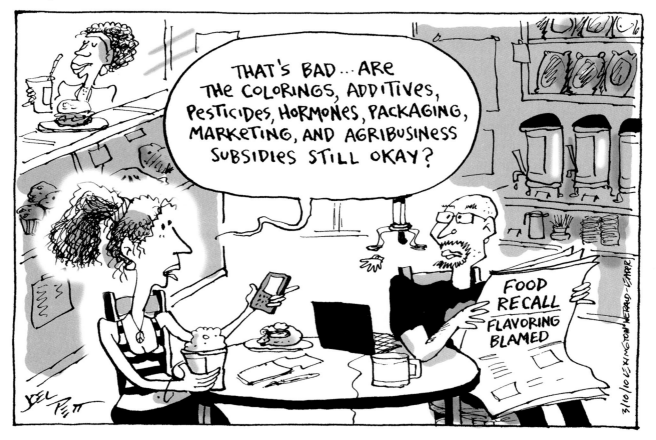

The uncertainties derive from the scientific complexities of studying chemicals that are consumed in small amounts— parts per million, billion, or trillion. Larger amounts of pesticides are demonstrably harmful to farmworkers. It may be difficult to believe that even smaller amounts can possibly be good for human health, but their long-term effects are not well established. Consumers cannot easily avoid these chemicals, and their amounts in common foods are rarely known unless advocacy groups measure them. ▶

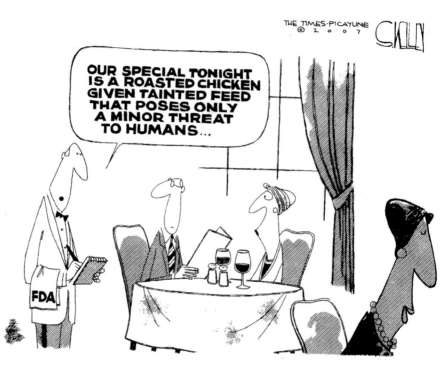

Like GMOs and cloning, pesticide levels are not disclosed on food labels. ▼

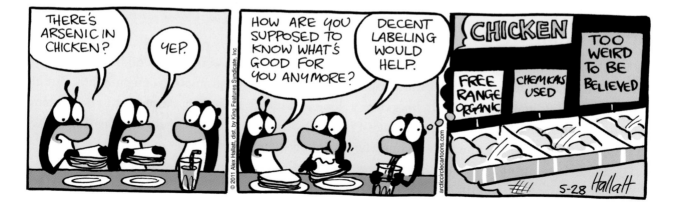

BISPHENOL A (BPA) IN BABY BOTTLES

Among chemical contaminants in foods, bisphenol A (BPA) elicits the most concern. BPA is a component of a hard, type-7 polycarbonate plastic used to make baby bottles and to line food cans. But it is an endocrine disrupter that mimics the actions of estrogen. Of the great many studies that have examined its effects, some show links to neurological problems and cancer, while others do not. The FDA says that BPA is safe at current levels of exposure but has banned its use in baby bottles. ▼

BPA highlights the divide between two approaches to safety regulation: precautionary ("if it might be bad, keep it out of the food supply until proven safe") and laissez-faire ("leave it in the food supply until proven harmful"). In the case of BPA, the FDA plays it both ways. Canada, however, has banned it.

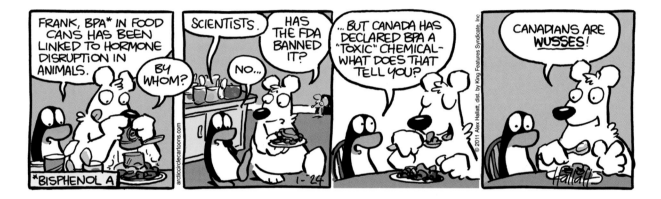

METHYLMERCURY IN FISH

In *What to Eat,* I described the presence of toxic mercury in fish as creating a dilemma: Fish are good to eat for their nutritional value and especially for their health-promoting omega-3 fats. But all seafood is contaminated with methylmercury, a toxic substance especially damaging to developing fetuses during the early months of pregnancy. Pregnant women must take care to avoid eating highly contaminated fish, but too much methylmercury is not good for anyone. ◤

The methylmercury that gets into seafood comes from mercury emitted by volcanoes, but it also comes from industrial pollution. Once in water, mercury is transformed into methylmercury and

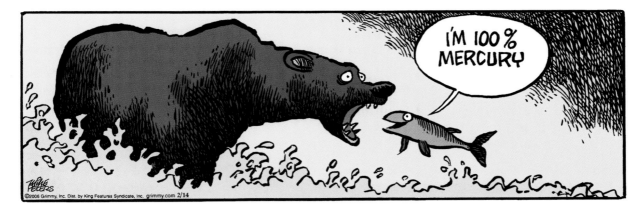

incorporated into algae. Little fish eat algae. Big fish eat little fish. Methylmercury accumulates in fish muscle tissue as it moves up the food chain, so its greatest food sources are large predatory fish: sharks, swordfish, king mackerel, tilefish, and albacore (white) tuna.

What to do? The mercury-in-seafood problem illustrates the difference between dietary interventions focused on public health and those focused on personal responsibility. We could turn off or clean the emissions from coal-burning power plants so fish are less contaminated in the first place. But industrial producers much prefer to leave it up to you to protect yourself. To avoid methylmercury, you have to know the difference between one fish and another, how much methylmercury each contains, and how much fish you are allowed to eat—rather a lot for most eaters and restaurant employees to master. ▲

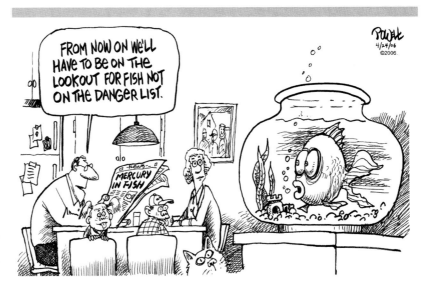

OIL IN GULF SEAFOOD

Mercury is not the only safety problem for seafood. In 2010, a deep oil well owned by BP (British Petroleum) had a blowout in the Gulf of Mexico and leaked great volumes of oil for months before it could be capped. This caused an ecological disaster. Supplies of local seafood were damaged by the oil itself as well as by the resulting lack of oxygen and the chemical dispersants used to remove the oil. ▼

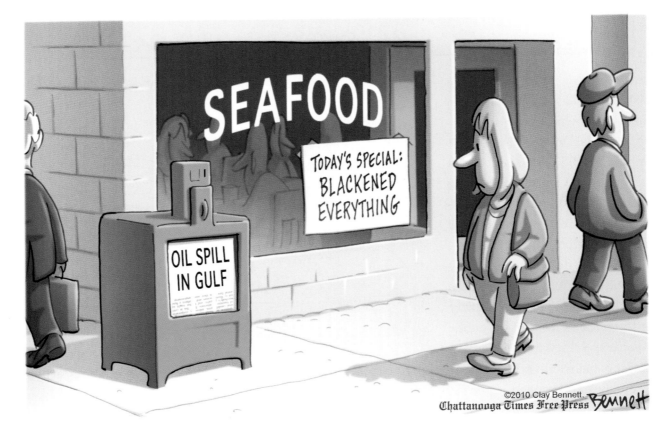

©2010 Clay Bennett. *Chattanooga Times Free Press* BENNETT

New Orleans shrimp fishers, still reeling from the effects of Hurricane Katrina in 2005, were not permitted to fish or sell their products for weeks. At one point, the FDA came in and pronounced Gulf shrimp safe to eat. How did the FDA determine safety? By nose. The agency trained 40 inspectors to sniff out traces of oil on the shrimp. ▼

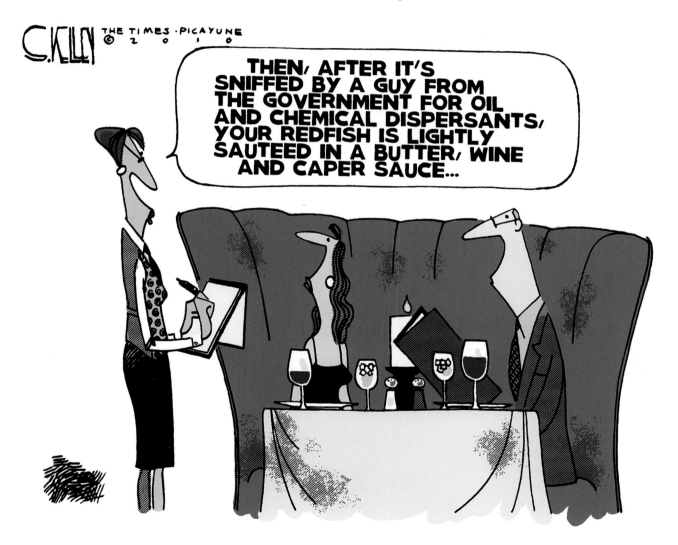

RADIOACTIVITY IN FISH FROM JAPAN

In March 2011, a powerful earthquake and subsequent tsunami swept over Japan. Along with much other devastation, it caused a partial meltdown in the Fukushima Daiichi nuclear power plant and the consequent release of radioactive particles into the atmosphere. Within short order, Japanese officials identified increasing levels of radioactive elements in plankton, small fish and shellfish, and eventually in larger fish. How serious a health problem did this pose for American consumers? The FDA did extensive testing of seafood samples and said none were of concern, especially in comparison to other health hazards. But such an answer is hardly reassuring. ▶▶

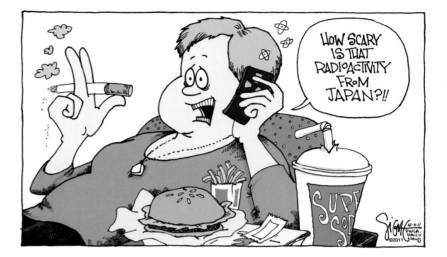

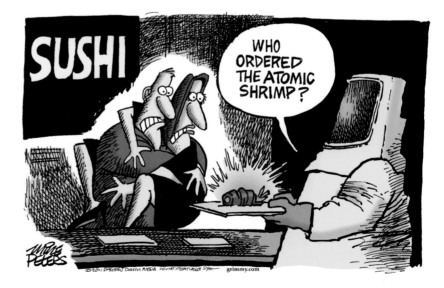

MOST FRIGHTENING OF ALL: MAD COW DISEASE

I FIRST LEARNED about mad cow disease in the mid-1990s when it caused a crisis in Great Britain. The disease had affected at least 175,000 cows, caused more than four million cattle to be slaughtered, generated costs estimated at $7 billion, been transmitted to at least 18 countries, and resulted in worldwide rejection of British beef. By the early 2000s, mad cow disease had caused at least 120 human deaths. ▼

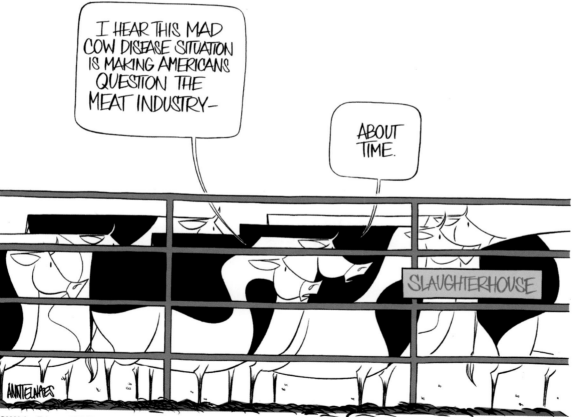

Mad cow disease (more formally, bovine spongiform encephalopathy or BSE) is especially worrying because it is caused by a bizarre infectious agent: prions. These are misformed protein particles that destroy the brain and nervous system and are invariably fatal. Prions cause cows to behave strangely. Such particles also are responsible for scrapies in sheep and related diseases in other animals.

The most likely initial cause of the British mad cow disaster was the feeding of inadequately rendered offal from scrapies-infected sheep to cows, and reinforcement by feeding offal from diseased cows to other cows. Prions are extremely difficult to destroy, as they resist heat and digestive enzymes. To prevent mad cow disease, cows must not be fed offal containing parts of animal nervous systems. Because prion diseases can occur spontaneously, prevention also means keeping older cows and "downer" cows (those that can't walk) out of the food supply. It helps to test for prion diseases, too. But all of these preventive measures are expensive for the beef industry. ◄

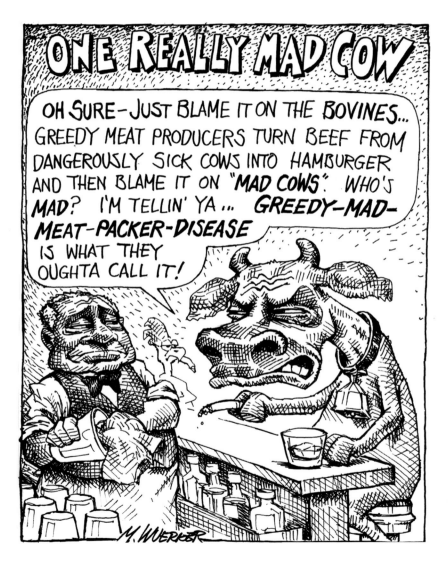

In the United States, federal agencies ban animal proteins in feed for ruminant animals. They also ban imports of rendered animal products from countries that cannot prove their cattle are free of the disease. Food safety officials say the virtual absence of mad cow disease and its human variant in the United States is due to such preventive actions. But "virtual" is in the eye of the beholder. Since testing began, officials have identified four cows with BSE in the United States, one each in 2003, 2004, and 2006, and 2012. These were all older cows. Because they were identified in advance, they never entered the food supply. ▼

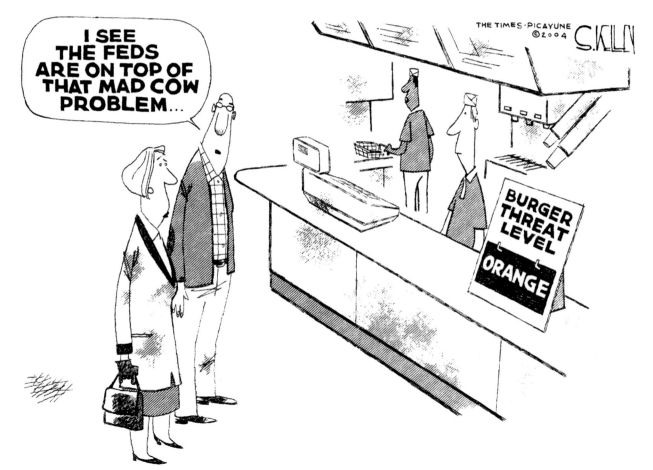

But could others have slipped through? The cow that tested positive for BSE in 2003 set off a panic. Beef exports and sales fell drastically. As a result, the USDA tested nearly 800,000 cows for BSE. When it identified only two cases, the beef industry celebrated, and the USDA greatly reduced the testing program. But without testing, can we be sure that beef is safe? ▼

In 2008, an employee of the Humane Society infiltrated a slaughterhouse owned by Hallmark/Westland Beef Packing and secretly filmed the slaughter of "downer" cows for food as well as other violations of USDA rules. Because downer cows are at high risk for BSE, the company had to recall more than 143 million pounds of raw and frozen beef products, much of them destined for federal school meals and emergency feeding programs. This event, to say the least, raised questions about

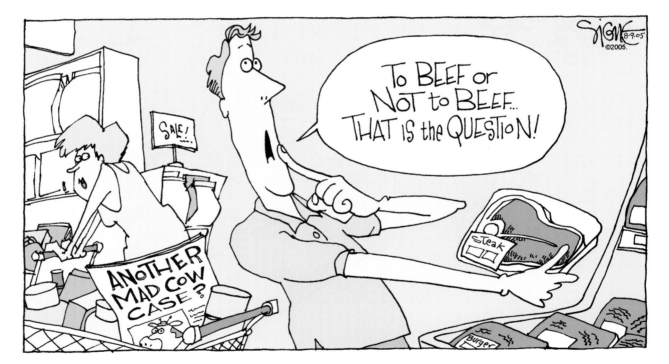

the USDA's ability to adequately monitor meat safety and about what consumers, as individuals, would have to do to protect themselves. ▼ ▼

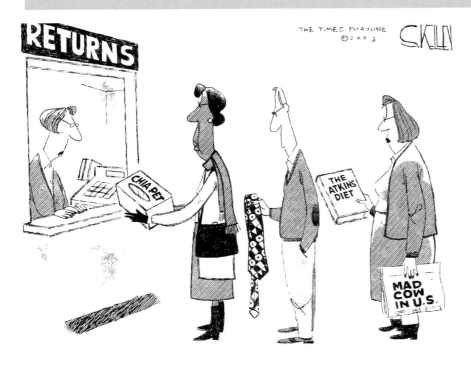

Would having better oversight of food safety prevent mad cow and other problems? I think so. And so would having a food safety system that unites the oversight functions of USDA and FDA. But that goal, at the moment, is unlikely to be politically feasible.

8

Food Labels versus Marketing

ANY EXCURSION INTO A SUPERMARKET TAKES you to aisles filled with food products laden with sugars, saturated fats, salt, and excess calories, all heavily promoted and highly profitable for makers and sellers, if not for the people who eat them. In many stores, entire aisles are devoted to sodas, snack foods, cookies, candy, and sugary breakfast cereals. These foods are made with inexpensive ingredients, advertised with enormous budgets, and manufactured by some of the largest food corporations in the world.

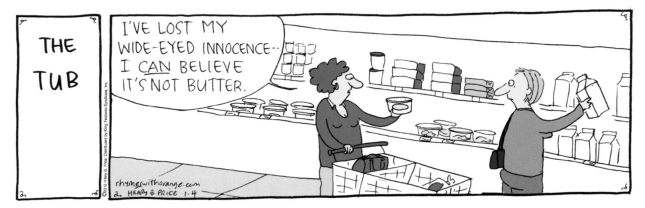

Food manufacturers and retailers say that processed foods give you what you want and need: easy-to-eat foods that require little preparation and taste better than anything you could make yourself. Maybe, but most of these products are processed foods of minimal nutritional value—"junk foods"—filled with texturizers, colors, and flavors designed to make them look and taste like "real" foods. ▲

Many of the ingredients are preservatives added to extend shelf life, thereby enabling manufacturers to buy ingredients when prices are low and sell the products at hefty profits. ▼

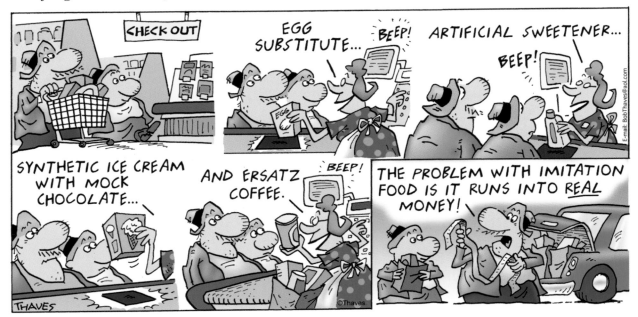

Old Name: **Beef Jerky**

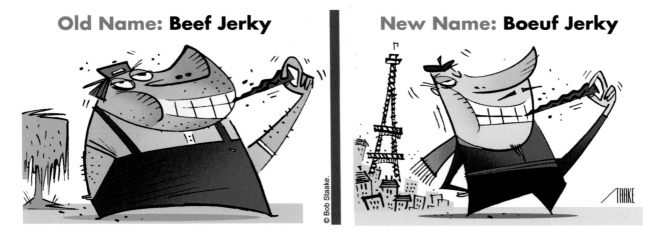

New Name: **Boeuf Jerky**

©2007 baloocartoons.com

Creating and marketing processed food products takes imagination and skill. What foods are called, for example, can have an important influence on sales. ▲

But marketers who overly market the attributes of their foods are taking a risk. If the products don't deliver on promises, customers will stop buying them. ▶

The marketers of junk foods are fortunate: They have human nature on their side. People typically believe that healthful foods cannot possibly

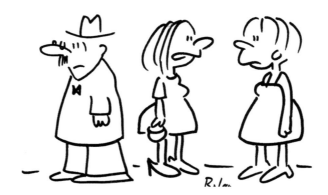

"I'VE FED HIM PAUL NEWMAN SALAD DRESSING, PAUL NEWMAN SPAGHETTI SAUCE, AND PAUL NEWMAN POPCORN, BUT NONE OF IT DOES ANY GOOD!"

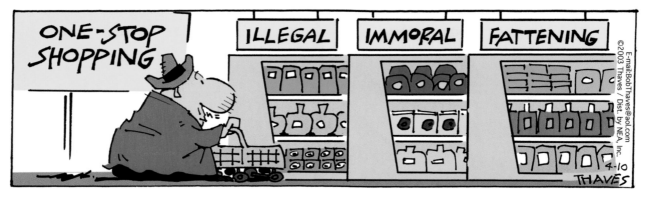

taste good and that anything delicious is undoubtedly bad for health. ▲

Much research has gone into explaining the basis of food marketing. Researchers find, for example, that emphasizing the positive attributes of a food is often more effective than focusing on the negative—the bad things that the food might do to you. ▼

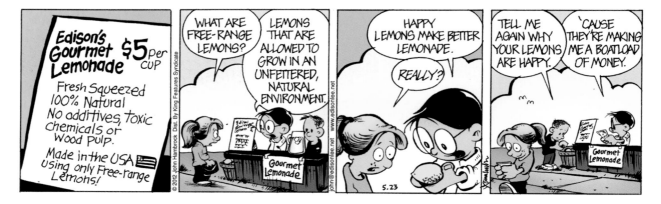

Customers may say they want to eat healthfully, but many people are confused by nutrition advice and complicated ingredient lists. Marketers take advantage of this confusion. ▼ ▼

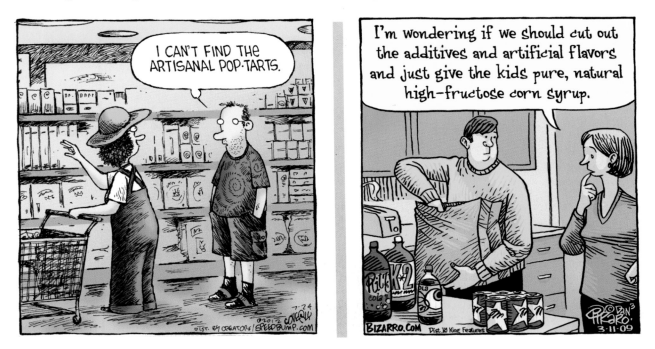

Food marketers, of course, are always looking for ways to cut costs and increase profits. ▼

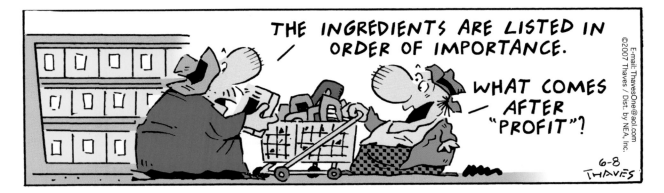

Because price is a strong determinant of consumer food choice, manufacturers look for ways to respond to rising ingredient costs that do not involve price increases. They may, for example, reduce package sizes but keep prices constant. This might work—unless customers notice it. ▼

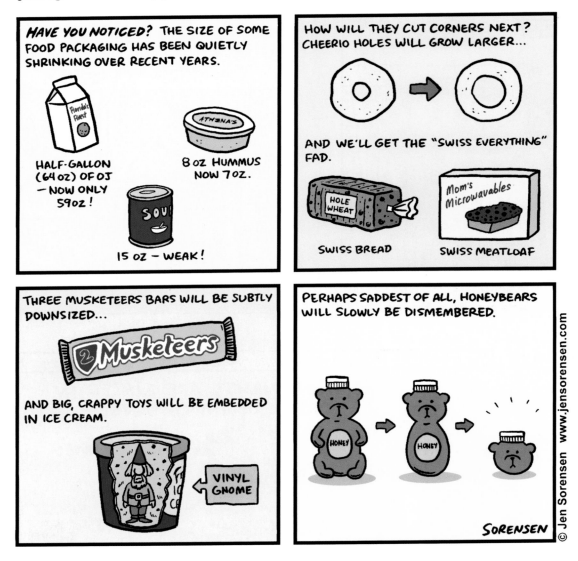

INFORMING CUSTOMERS: FOOD LABELS

TO HELP THE PUBLIC contend with misleading marketing, Congress passed the Nutrition Labeling and Education Act of 1990. This act instituted the current labeling system. Congress intended the new label to perform multiple functions:

- Reveal the calories, nutrients, and ingredients in food products
- Discourage consumption of fat, saturated fat, cholesterol, and sodium (and, later, trans fat)
- Encourage consumption of "problem" nutrients—vitamin A, vitamin C, calcium, iron, and fiber
- Permit comparison to daily needs

The FDA dealt with these requirements by designing a two-part label—Nutrition Facts and the ingredient list—so difficult to understand that a lengthy, color-coded Web site complete with self-guided tests is needed to explain it. ▲

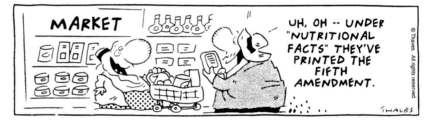

The Nutrition Facts panel is difficult to understand at best, but especially so when manufacturers deliberately use it to mislead consumers. ▼

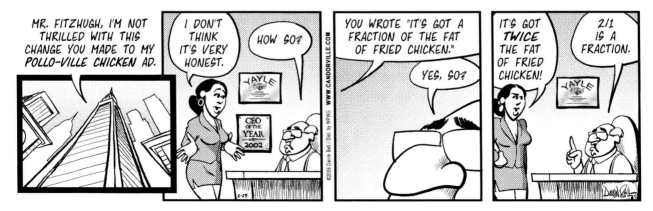

The least understood part of the Nutrition Facts panel has to do with serving size. The FDA established serving size standards for foods and beverages for use on food labels, but these are invariably smaller than what many people are accustomed to eating. If a package contains more than one serving, the nutrition information must be multiplied accordingly, but not every reader may remember to do this.

FDA regulations require food and beverage manufacturers to provide information about specific ingredients in their foods, in order of prominence. ▶▼

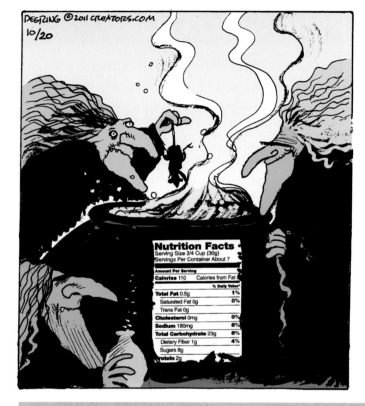

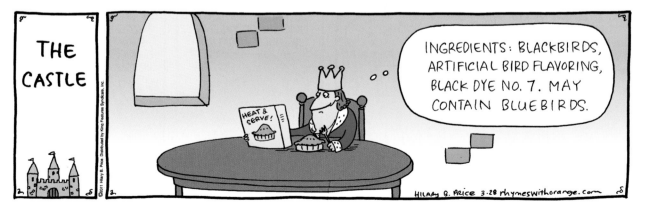

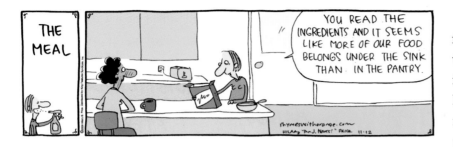

But from the beginning, food and beverage manufacturers were concerned that information in the Nutrition Facts panel and ingredient list might discourage sales of their products. ◀

LABELING BEVERAGES

A NUTRITION FACTS LABEL for water displays nothing but zeros. Its ingredient list contains one item: water. Unless manufacturers add things to it, water has no calories or nutrients. ▼

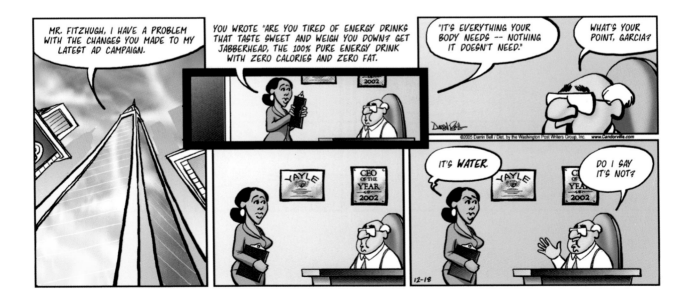

From a business standpoint, water poses a serious problem. It comes out of a tap and costs practically nothing. Putting it in bottles, however, allows it to be sold at a phenomenal profit. ▼

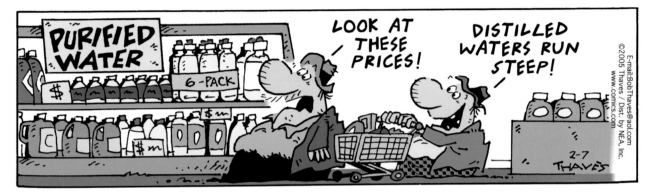

The addition of artificial sweeteners—aspartame, for example—to sweeten water permitted the creation of a diet soda industry able to market its products as calorie-free. But these products seem anything but natural, and their health effects are endlessly debated. ▼

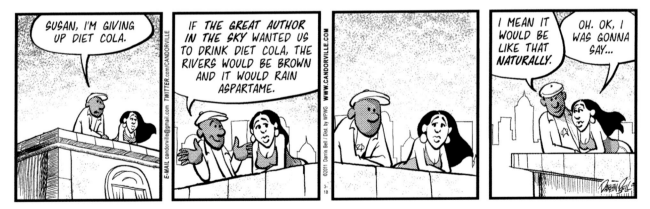

MARKETING HEALTH: LABEL CLAIMS

THE FOOD INDUSTRY spends billions of dollars a year to encourage people to buy their products, but foods marketed as "healthy" particularly encourage sales and, therefore, greater calorie intake. According to Cornell Professor Brian Wansink, people are likely to eat more calories from snack foods when they are labeled "low-fat," "no trans fat," or "organic." Most people, he says, are blissfully unaware of how the food environment influences what they eat. People take in excessive calories "not because of hunger but because of family and friends, packages and plates, names and numbers, labels and lights, colors and candles, shapes and smells. . . . The list is almost as endless as it's invisible."

NUTRIENT CONTENT CLAIMS

The nutrition labeling act specifies how the FDA must regulate claims made on food packages for nutrition and health benefits. These rules were needed because food manufacturers want to be able to promote the benefits of what's good in their products— the "eat more" ingredients— and deflect attention from the "eat less" ones. ▶ ▶

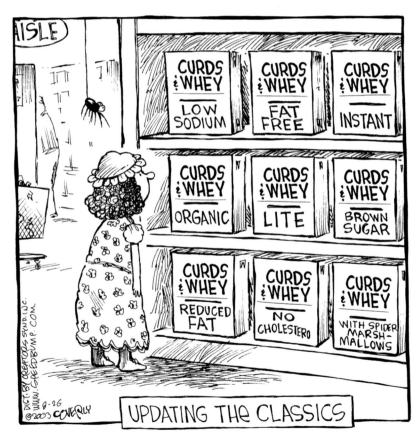

UPDATING THE CLASSICS

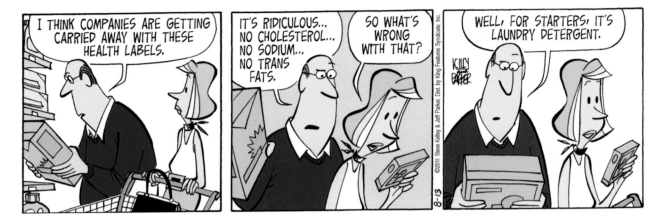

In recent years, one food company after another has dealt with health concerns by developing icons to identify the healthier, "better-for-you" options in their product lines. Because so many companies invented their own schemes for doing this, it became difficult to know what they meant. ▶

Some of my more conspiracy-minded colleagues think the FDA deliberately designed the Nutrition Facts label to be confusing, but I see it more as the result of inevitable compromises. You want to know what is in the foods you buy, but food companies are afraid that you will use the label to classify foods as good or bad. So the Nutrition Facts label tells you what Congress said it had to, as interpreted by the FDA, under pressure from vested interests. The result: a design that confuses more than it helps.

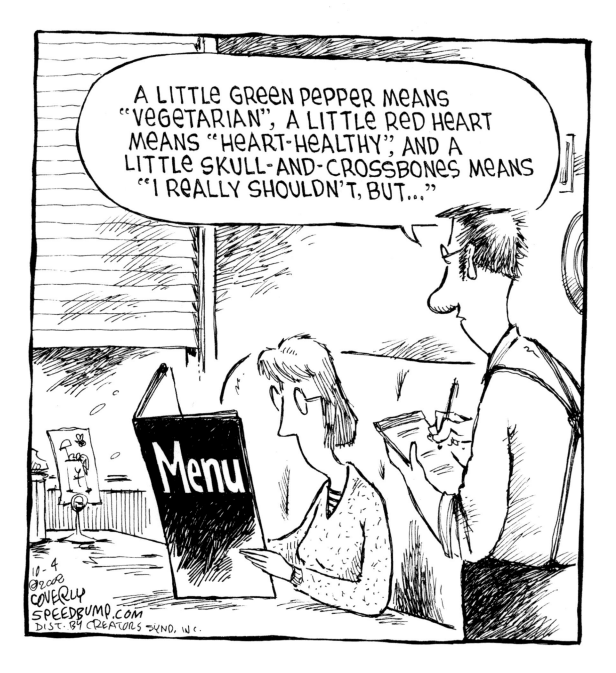

9 Fixing the Food System: Regulations

WHETHER AND HOW MUCH THE GOVERNMENT should be involved in the food choices of individual citizens is a matter of ongoing public debate. For public health, putting some limits on food industry marketing practices is a good idea because such limits make it easier for people to make healthier food choices. But people holding other points of view do not want the government dictating personal dietary choices, especially when such choices cause no harm to anyone but themselves. ▶

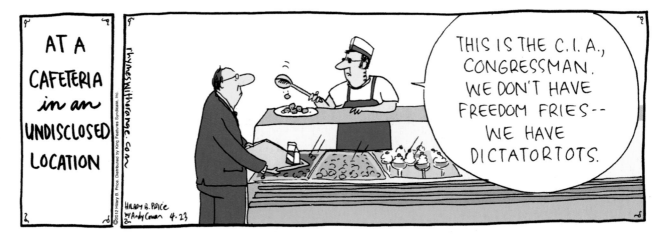

They argue that the government should stay out of such seemingly trivial matters as the salt intake of individuals or misleading health claims on food packages. ▼ ▶

Driving the current version of this debate is what to do about the rising prevalence of obesity, a problem certain to increase the cost of health care to taxpayers. The argument for government intervention is based on research showing how profoundly the food marketing environment influences personal dietary choices. By setting limits on marketing practices, governments can encourage healthier choices, help prevent obesity and its consequences, and reduce health care costs.

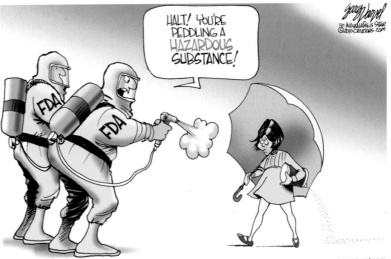

garyvarvel.com

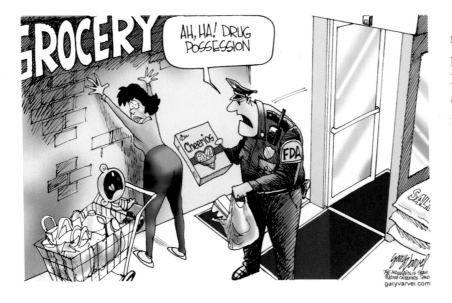

Furthermore, the government *already* is involved in personal dietary choices. Federal policies support the current food environment, for example, by subsidizing the ingredients in processed foods, permitting corporations to deduct the cost of marketing from taxes as business expenses, and allowing junk foods to be marketed during children's television programs. Regulations to improve the food environment break no new ground. They merely tweak existing policies to promote health rather than illness.

This rationale has led city, state, and federal governments to seek ways to promote better food choices. New York City, for example, introduced a series of measures to ban trans fats, put calories on the menus of fast-food restaurants, tax sodas, and cap the size of sodas sold within city limits. Because such measures directly confront beliefs that government should stay out of personal choices, they are controversial and often elicit substantial pushback, as shown in these next examples.

BANNING TRANS FATS

TRANS FATS ARE AN easy target for intervention. They are artificially produced through partial hydrogenation of vegetable oils, are unnatural, and raise the risk of heart disease as much as or even more than saturated fats. Trans fats affect obesity only indirectly—healthier fats have as many calories. But they are a marker for junk food. And because removing them from the food supply is feasible, they have become a focal point of advocacy for changes in the food environment. ▼

In 2003, the FDA required trans fats to be listed on Nutrition Facts labels. That rule went into effect in 2006, but did not apply to restaurants and bakeries. Restaurant owners like using partially hydrogenated oils because they are cheap—soybean production is subsidized—and have a long shelf life.

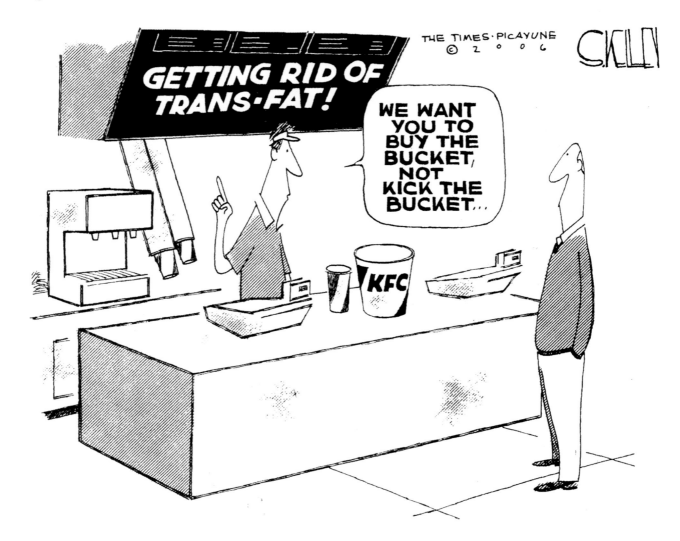

In 2005, the New York City Board of Health, concerned about high rates of heart disease among residents, asked restaurant owners to voluntarily replace hydrogenated cooking oils with healthier oils. Few complied, mainly because owners did not understand the difference between one kind of cooking oil and another. A year later, the board voted to restrict use of "unhealthful artificial trans fats" in all of the city's food service establishments. ▼

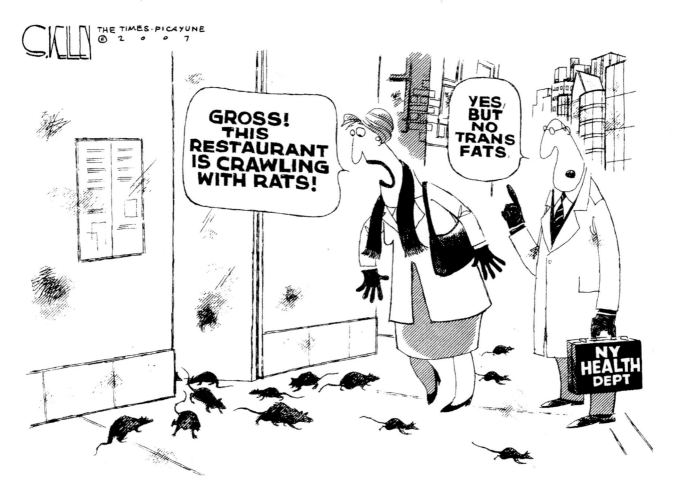

The ban surprised observers who see food as nowhere near as harmful as cigarettes. Some thought that the city had gone too far. ▶

But studies show that restaurants are now using healthier oils and New Yorkers are consuming less trans fat to the greater good of their health. Trans fats, however, are only one of several dietary components that adversely affect health, and the extent to which this ban will reduce heart disease remains to be determined. ▼

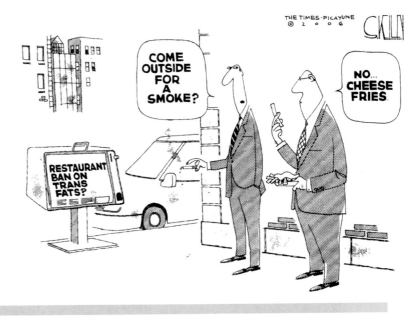

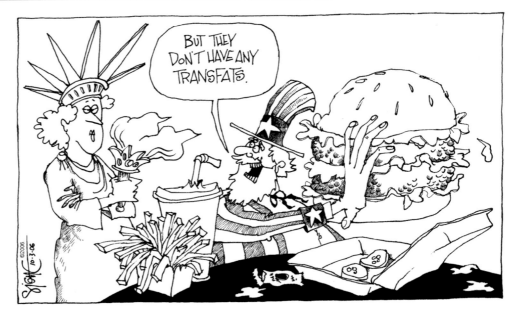

POSTING CALORIES

FREQUENT CONSUMPTION of fast food raises the risk for obesity. Fast food and sugar-sweetened beverages are highly caloric, especially when super-sized. Because their calories are accompanied by no or relatively few nutrients, they are considered "empty." Products with empty, or relatively empty calories, constitute "junk foods." ▶

In 2008, New York City began to require fast-food and chain restaurants to post the number of calories in each item on menu boards. Other cities soon instituted their own rules, but these were so inconsistent that the National Restaurant Association eventually stopped fighting the idea and instead supported enactment of a national law to

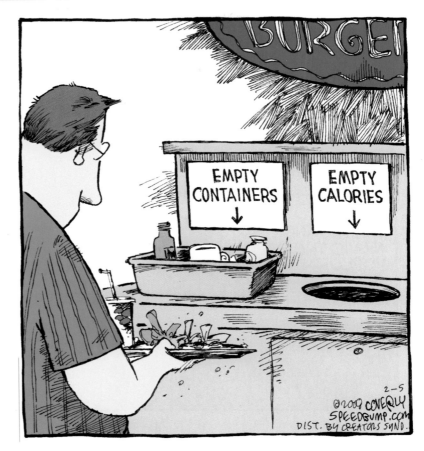

preempt local initiatives. In the way such things work, Congress inserted a mandate for menu labeling into the Affordable Care Act (the act that reformed health care). President Obama signed this into law in 2010. That mandate requires restaurants, food retail chains, and vending machines with more than 20 units nationwide to post the number of calories in their products in a "clear and conspicuous manner" along with an average value for daily calorie needs—2,000 per day. ▶

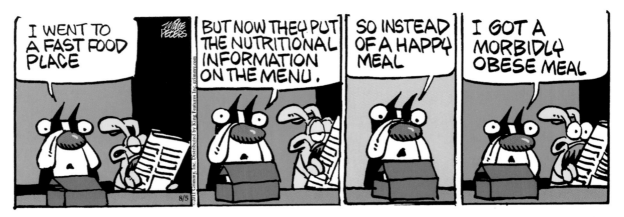

The FDA issued its first draft of the menu labeling rules in August 2010. These required calories to be posted for foods served in movie theaters, lunch wagons, bowling alleys, trains, and airlines. ▼

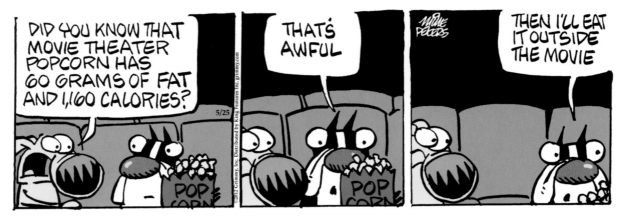

But one year later, when the FDA published proposed rules, it no longer required calorie labeling in these venues. The rules would not apply to businesses whose primary purpose is other than selling food. Because food is sold everywhere these days—drug, clothing, and business supply stores, for example—these exemptions undermine the purpose of menu labeling. An investigative report suggested that the White House had insisted on such exemptions out of fear of nanny-state complaints during a particularly contentious election year. In mid-2013, the FDA had yet to issue final rules for calorie labeling, and whether they would apply to movie theaters and other such venues was still uncertain.

TAXING JUNK FOODS AND SODAS

FOOD CHOICES ARE highly sensitive to price. Because low prices encourage sales and consumption, an obvious way to discourage purchases of unhealthful foods is to raise prices through taxes. But nobody likes being taxed, and it is not easy to mobilize popular support for this action. The food industry especially dislikes taxes or any other measures that might discourage sales. ▶

The easiest targets for tax strategies are sugar-sweetened beverages—sodas, juice drinks, and the like. Sodas contain sugars; they provide calories, but little or nothing else of nutritional value. Many people consume sodas in large volumes. Cutting down on soda consumption is an easy way to reduce calorie intake, but people who might most benefit from doing so are often those most opposed. ▶

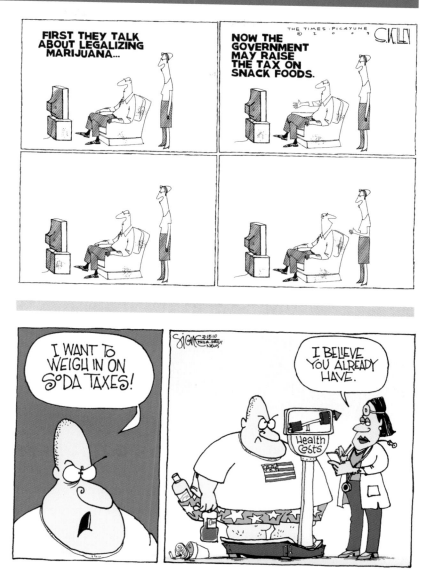

Soda taxes have one other benefit. They could provide badly needed revenue to local governments during an economic downturn. ▼

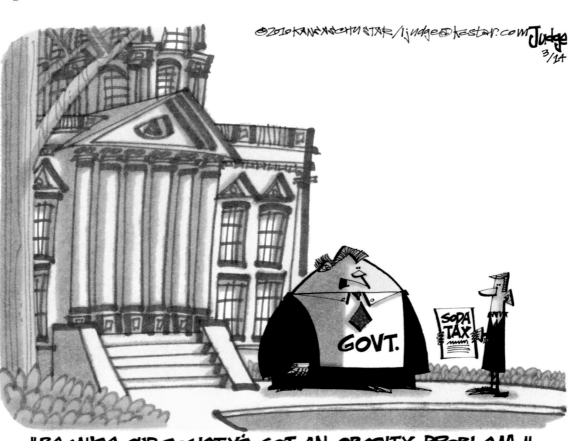

"BECAUSE OUR SOCIETY'S GOT AN OBESITY PROBLEM."

Despite their potential benefits, soda tax measures consistently fail to be enacted. Soda companies have lobbied fiercely—and successfully—against them. As of early 2013, at least 30 states had tried to tax sodas. All failed as a result of extensive lobbying and spending, said to have cost the soda industry $70 million or more.

CAPPING SODA SIZES

IN LATE MAY 2012, New York City's Mayor Michael Bloomberg announced that no sodas or sugary drinks larger than 16 ounces would be allowed to be sold in restaurants, movie theaters, and street carts within city limits. Health department studies indicated that more than half of New Yorkers were overweight or obese, with the greatest prevalence of obesity observed in neighborhoods where consumption of sodas was highest.

To public health advocates like me, a 16-ounce sugary drink seems generous. It constitutes *two* standard servings, includes nearly 50 grams of sugars—table sugar or high-fructose corn syrup—and provides about 200 "empty" (nutrient-free) calories. But others prefer to leave such matters to the food industry to decide, regardless of the effect of poor health on the cost of medical care. ▼ ▶

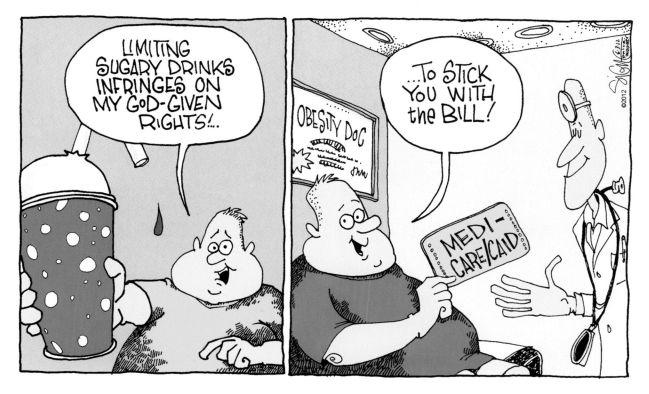

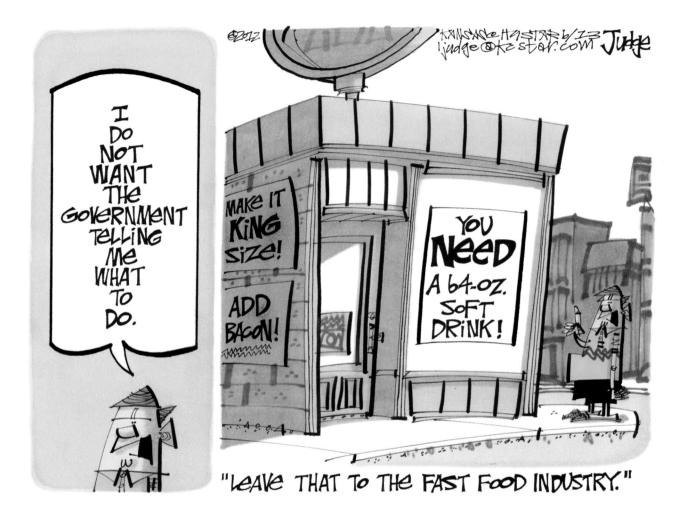

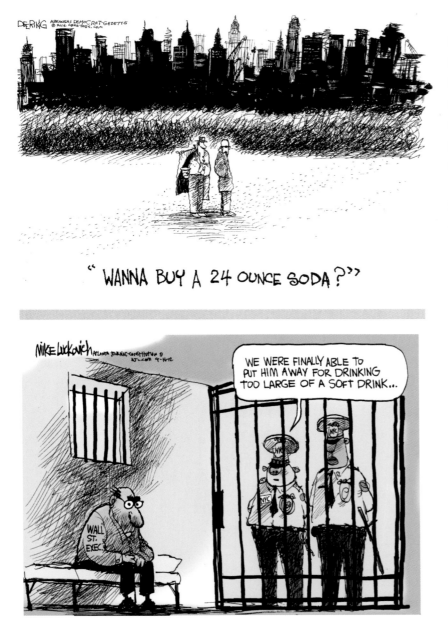

"WANNA BUY A 24 OUNCE SODA?"

WE WERE FINALLY ABLE TO PUT HIM AWAY FOR DRINKING TOO LARGE OF A SOFT DRINK...

Some opponents predicted that the soda cap, like Prohibition, would lead people to break the law to consume illegal-size drinks, giving authorities an excuse to jail people who had gotten away with much more serious crimes. ◀◀

In fighting the cap, the soda industry appealed directly to emotions about personal freedom: "Don't let bureaucrats tell you what size beverage soda to buy." The American Beverage Association funded a so-called grassroots ("Astroturf") pro-soda coalition, petitions, home mailings, truck posters, and billboards. In doing so, the soda industry was positioning itself as a self-interested promoter of poor diets and obesity while also drumming up antigovernment and anti–public health sentiments. When all else failed, the Beverage Association sued and succeeded in blocking the measure, at least temporarily.

THE FOOD INDUSTRY: RESPONDING TO CRITICS

FOOD COMPANIES HAVE responded to pressure from health advocates by attempting to "health up" their products, but doing so presents them with serious marketing challenges. ▶▶

A common food industry tactic to deflect attention from nutrition issues is to reformulate products to make them more environmentally friendly. ▶

For business reasons, companies cannot make health-promoting changes in ingredients if doing so reduces sales. This fundamental problem means that regulation is the intervention most likely to improve the food marketing environment.

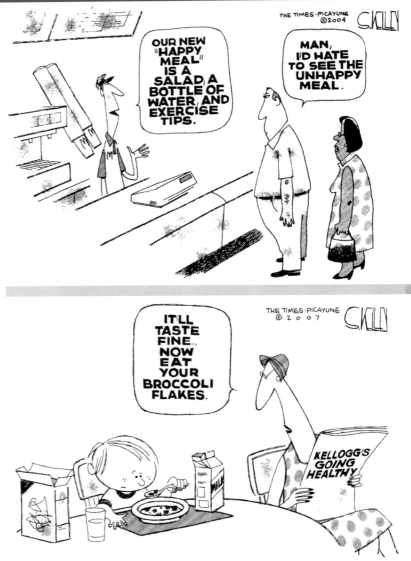

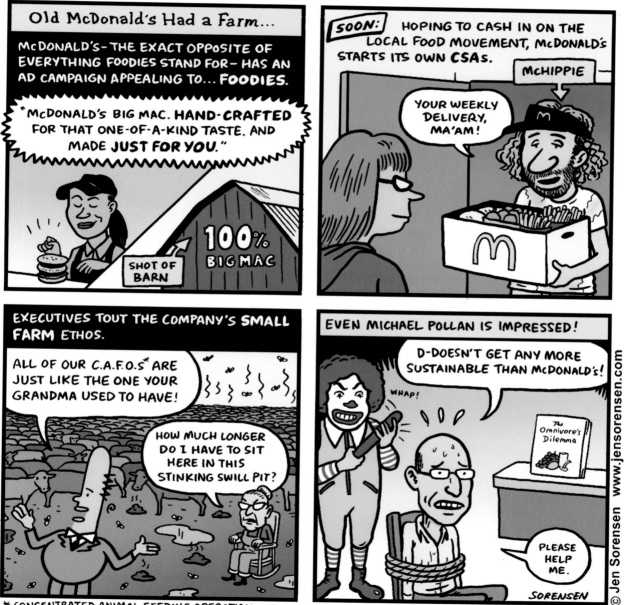

10 Fixing the Food System: The Food Movement

THAT THE CURRENT INDUSTRIAL FOOD SYSTEM needs fixing is best illustrated by its effects. Americans have access to a consistent, low-cost food supply almost entirely independent of season, weather, or geography.

But efficient and productive as it is, this system has some profoundly undesirable consequences. One is the loss of taste quality in foods bred for transportability and long shelf life rather than taste. ▶

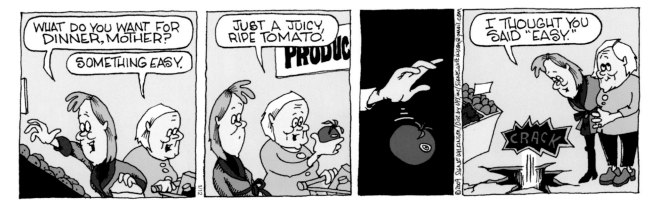

A more critical effect is on the world's climate. Industrial agriculture is estimated to account for a significant fraction of greenhouse gas emissions, largely because of methane gas produced by livestock, and carbon and other gas-forming emissions that occur during the manufacture and use of fertilizers, pesticides, and farm machinery. ▶

Although it might seem self-evident that the climate is getting warmer and weather more extreme, some people believe

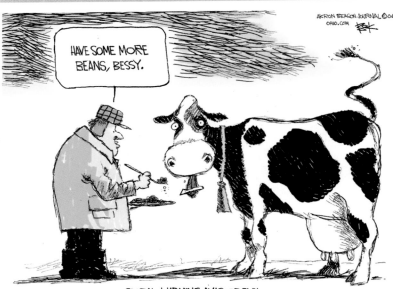

GLOBAL WARMING AXIS OF EVIL

that these trends do not have anything to do with human industrial or agricultural activity and that it is not necessary to try to reduce the impact of agriculture on climate.

But scientists view greenhouse gases as already at levels so high that damage to agricultural production is inevitable. They predict that global warming will lead to more frequent extreme weather conditions such as the drought that affected midwestern farming states in 2012. ▶ ▼

If politicians cannot commit to policies to reverse global warming, then ordinary citizens will have to take action. And they are, as witnessed by today's burgeoning food movement.

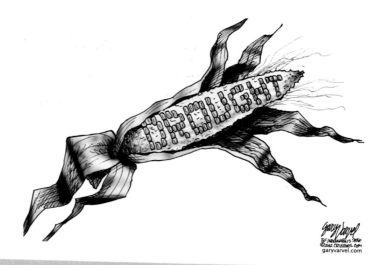

Tea Party Still Refuses Global Warming Facts

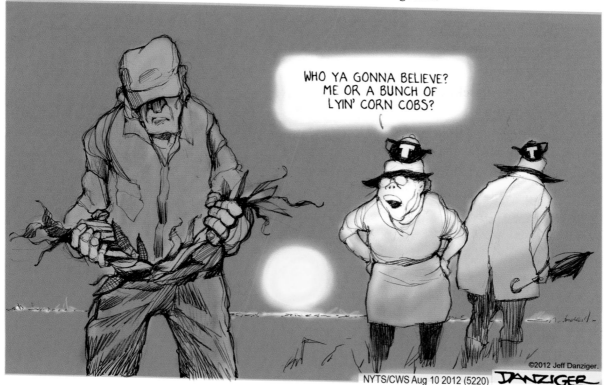

CHANGING THE FOOD SYSTEM

DESPITE PERSONAL AND environmental barriers to healthful eating, Americans are in the midst of a nation-wide social movement focused on improving the food system. This movement is fragmented and decentralized, composed of hundreds of genuine grassroots groups working for better health, food security, obesity prevention, and food safety, among other issues discussed in this book. Many groups want to transform industrial food production into a system that is more sustainable, local, and organic; kinder to farm animals; and fair and just to farmworkers. One common goal unites food movement groups: creating a food system that is healthier for people and the planet. Participants in this movement vote with their forks every time they make a food choice. ▲

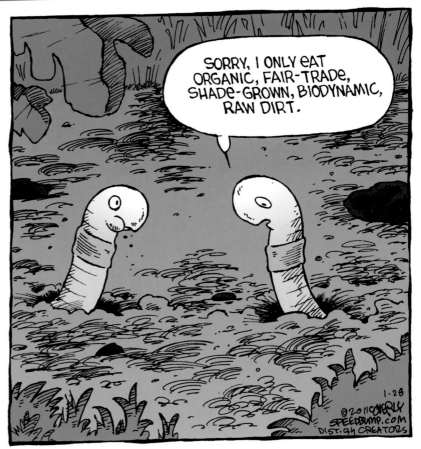

For people who view such issues as matters of personal choice and responsibility, or who simply are pressed for time, the various components of the movement may appear unrealistic and elitist. ▼ ▼

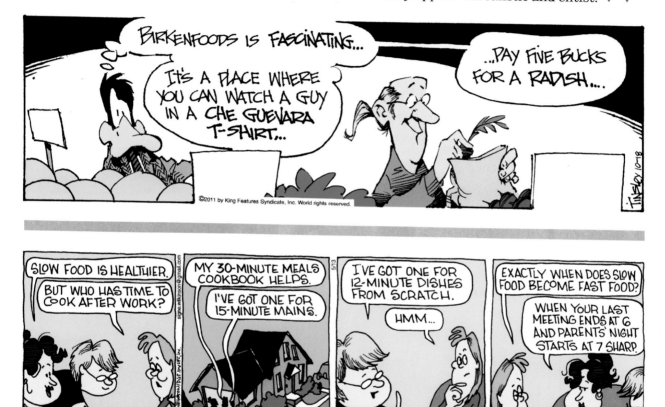

Even for active participants in the movement, putting principles into practice can lead to difficult conversations in restaurants and, sometimes, at home. ▼ ▼

BUYING LOCAL

THE MOVEMENT TO BUY LOCAL is so widespread that practitioners are now known as locavores. Food produced nearby is fresher—it doesn't have to travel thousands of miles to appear in supermarkets weeks after harvest—and it tastes better. Because locally grown food

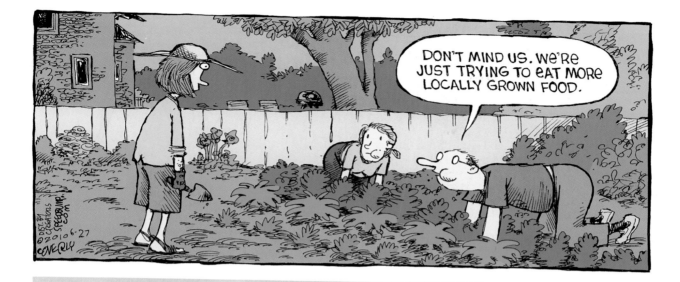

requires less transportation and storage, it can be kinder to the environment. ▲

Like most aspects of the food movement, the locavore movement can elicit skepticism, mainly because subsisting on locally grown food is inconvenient in cities, and advocates can sometimes seem unrealistically rigid. ▶ ▶

But most locavores I know are anything but extreme. They like the idea of supporting regional farmers and meeting them personally at farmers' markets. Most eat locally when it's convenient but don't even try for 100 percent. Buying just a few foods from local farmers helps them make a living and creates a more vibrant and cohesive community.

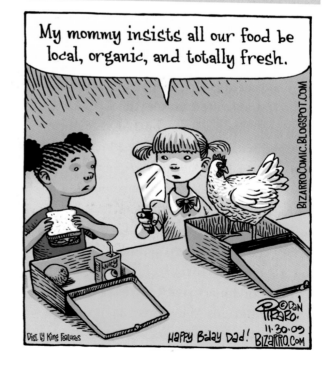

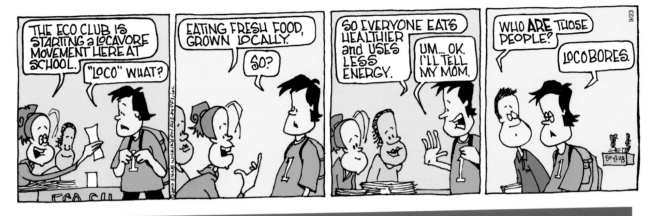

The Eco Club is starting a locavore movement here at school.

"Loco" what?

Eating fresh food, grown locally.

So?

So everyone eats healthier and uses less energy.

Um... Ok. I'll tell my mom.

Who **ARE** those people?

Locobores.

BUYING ORGANIC

ORGANIC FOODS CONSTITUTE one of the fastest-growing segments of the food industry, driven in part because they provide an option for people who want to avoid pesticides or genetically modified foods. In the United States, the USDA sets standards for foods permitted to display the Certified Organic seal.

To qualify for organic certification, the producers of organic fruits, vegetables, and grains may not use synthetic pesticides, herbicides, or fertilizers. ▶

They may not plant genetically modified seeds, use fertilizer derived from sewage sludge, or treat the seeds or foods with irradiation. They must keep records of everything they use and submit to

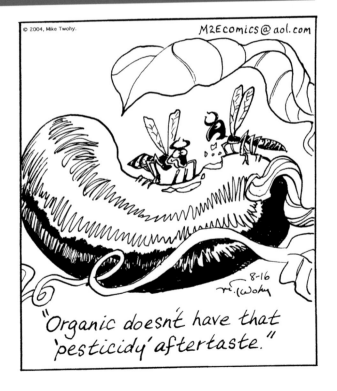

© 2004, Mike Twohy.   M2EcOMICS@aol.com

"Organic doesn't have that 'pesticidy' aftertaste."

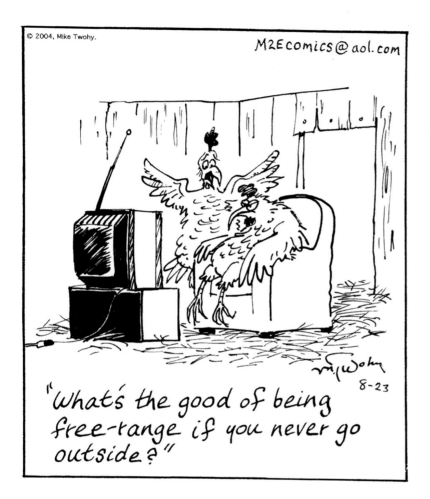

M2ECOMICS @ aol.com

"What's the good of being free-range if you never go outside?"

unannounced inspection by a USDA-accredited state or private certification agency. Producers of certified organic meats and poultry are not allowed to feed their animals by-products derived from other animals, may not use antibiotics and hormones, and must raise their animals and birds under conditions somewhat more humane than those typical of industrial feedlots and henhouses. These are all good reasons for people to buy organic foods.

The standards—the rules about what organic farmers can and cannot do—are lengthy and do not make light reading. Like any set of rules, they have loopholes. The rules for organic egg production, for example, require that hens have access to the outdoors, but for a long time did not require that they actually *be* outdoors (that loophole has now been closed, at least in part). ▲

Opponents of organics—and there are many—work hard to make consumers doubt the reliability of organic certification. They also try to weaken the organic standards (so there really will be something

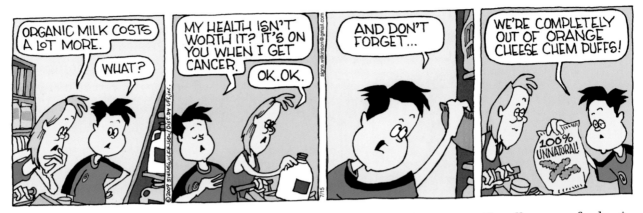

to doubt) and question whether organics are any better for you than conventionally grown foods. ▲

Driving this critique is the enormous success of the organic industry. Organic foods and beverages accounted for $29 billion in US sales in 2011. Organic foods generally cost more than mass-produced industrial food. Many people—out of preference or necessity—view the price of food as the paramount determinant of their choices. For them, organic prices are prohibitive. ▼

For others, however, the benefits in taste and production values are well worth the price.

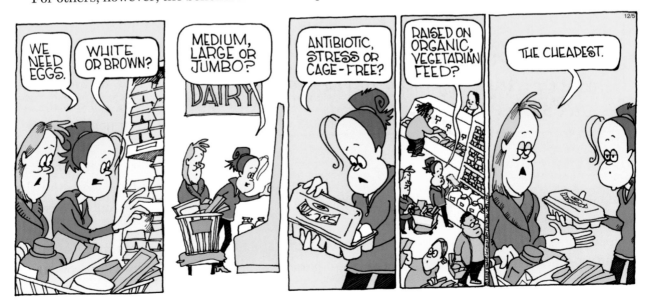

PROTECTING ANIMAL WELFARE

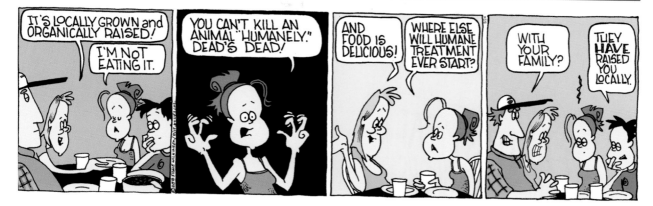

PEOPLE WHO EAT MEAT must come to terms with an unpleasant reality: Cows and chickens must die that we may live. ▲

The animal welfare movement attracts participants ranging from those who want more humane living conditions for livestock and chickens to those who would completely abolish raising animals for food. The more activist elements of this movement insist on enforcing humane standards of animal welfare, even going so far as to engage in rescue operations. ▼

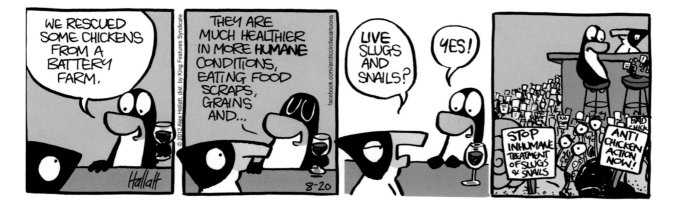

Meat eaters may well disagree with the basic premises of the animal welfare movement, but its adherents point to significant advantages of eating less or no meat: better health for people and less damage to the environment. ▼

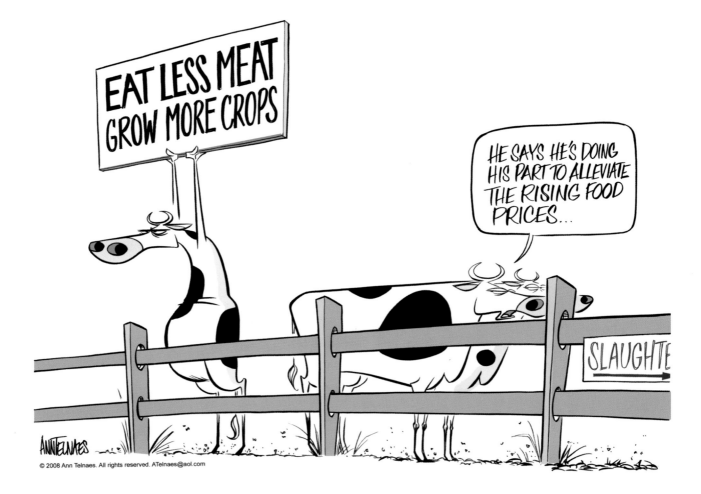

CHOOSING TO GO VEGETARIAN

VEGETARIANS FOLLOW A variety of dietary practices that share a partial or complete reliance on foods of plant origin. Some vegetarians will eat dairy products (lacto-vegetarians), eggs (ovo-vegetarians), fish (pescatarians), or poultry in addition to food plants. Vegans are vegetarians who eat no animal products whatsoever. The one common feature of vegetarian diets is avoidance of red meat, but some vegetarians even waive this restriction at times. ▼

Vegetarians are demonstrably healthier as a group than are people who eat meat; their rates of obesity, heart disease, and certain cancers are below those of average Americans. ▼

As long as vegetarians eat any other animal product—dairy, fish, eggs, poultry—they can avoid eating meat without affecting the nutritional quality of their diets.

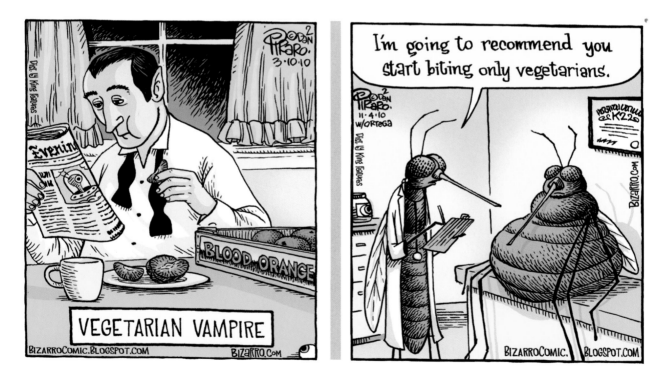

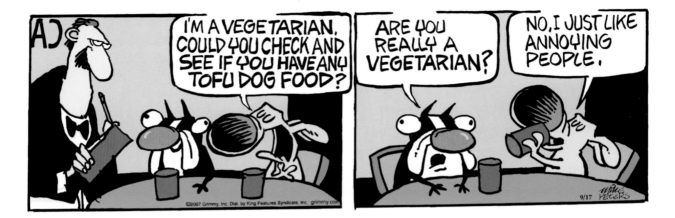

Vegans—who strictly avoid any foods of animal origin—do so for ethical as well as health and other reasons. ▼ Vegan diets, however, require some attention. ▲

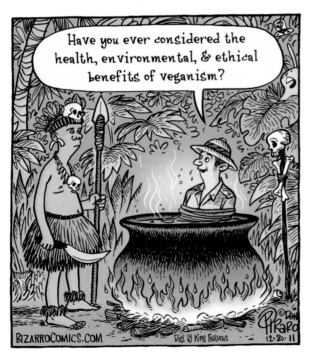

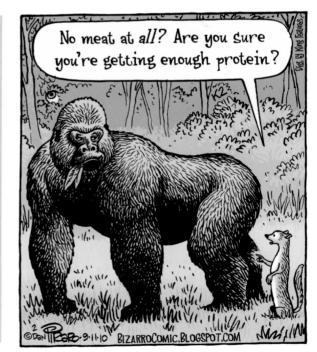

They must be sure to find an alternative source of vitamin B_{12} (the one vitamin found only in animal-based foods), to consume enough calories to maintain a healthy weight, and to eat a variety of grains and beans to get enough protein. ◣

GROWING THE FOOD MOVEMENT

ONE WAY TO DEAL with distress about the quality of industrial food is to grow your own. All over America, people are discovering that they can grow food practically anywhere. ▼

Really, all it takes to grow vegetables is some vacant land, sun, water, and a little knowledge of

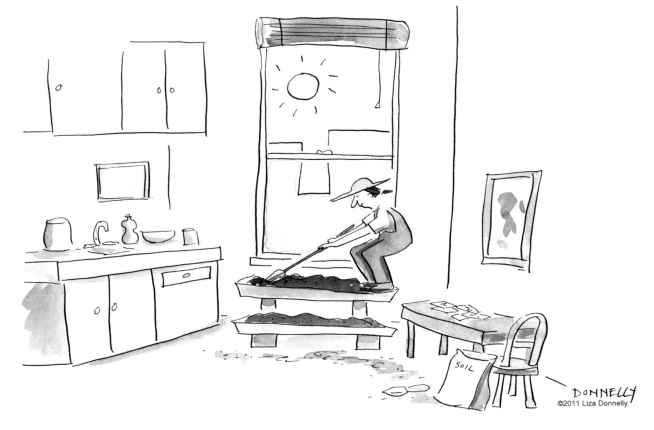

what plants need to grow. The gardening movement has been highly successful in introducing people to the farm-to-fork idea, but convincing them to want healthier foods is not always easy. ▼ ▼

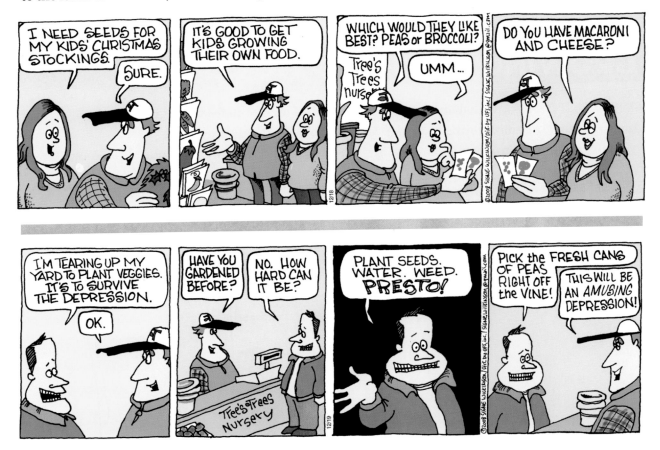

As should be evident by now, we are living in an era of grassroots political democracy organized around food issues. Today's food movement is expressed through advocacy for farmers' markets and local, seasonal, and sustainably produced food, and through resistance to corporate control of the food supply. Campaigns against childhood obesity and better school food—from sources no less than the White House—have raised awareness of food concerns and the need to improve the food system. Advocates are working to improve the quality of life for farmworkers and farm animals, and to reduce the impact of agriculture on climate change. Cartoonists are key contributors to this movement. May they flourish! ▼

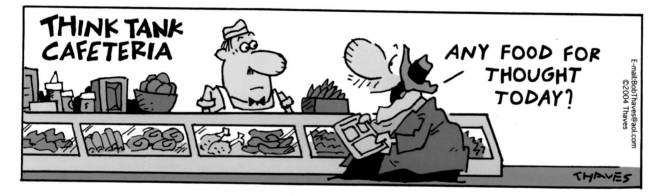

NOTES

INTRODUCTION

Page ix. The Senate inserted an amendment...: President Obama signed the Consolidated and Further Continuing Appropriations Act of 2012 on November 18, 2011, http://www.govtrack.us/congress/bills/112/hr2112. Section 743 of the act covers the tomato paste requirement. See also "Nutrition Standards in the National School Lunch and School Breakfast Programs," USDA Web site, January 26, 2012, http://www.fns.usda.gov/cnd/governance/legislation/nutritionstandards.htm.

Page xi. I started using them in my books...: The cartoons remained in *Food Politics* through a revised edition in 2007 and a 10th anniversary edition in 2013. *Pet Food Politics* also contains a cartoon by Steve Kelley.

Page xvi. Food is an enormous business...: "Food Expenditures: Overview," USDA Web site, October 1, 2012, http://www.ers.usda.gov/data-products/food-expenditures.aspx#26634.

CHAPTER 1

Page 2. It encompasses everyone who owns or works...: "Global Food Industry," USDA Web site, last modified May 31, 2012, http://www.ers.usda.gov/topics/international-markets-trade/global-food-markets/global-food-industry.aspx.

Page 6. The bill authorized payments to the owners...: Daniel Imhoff, *Food Fight: The Citizen's Guide to the Next Food and Farm Bill* (Healdsburg, CA: Watershed Media, 2012).

Page 8. More than 20 states passed "cheeseburger" bills...: Rebecca Turano, "Agricultural Disparagement Statutes: An Overview" (paper, Pennsylvania State University Dickinson School of Law, April 2010), http://law.psu.edu/_file/aglaw/Agricultural_Disparagement_Statutes_Rebecca_Turano.pdf.

Page 10. The influx of this anonymous "dark money"...: W. H. Wiist, "Citizens United, Public Health, and Democracy: The Supreme Court Ruling, Its Implications, and Proposed Action," *American Journal of Public Health* 101, no. 7 (July 2011): 1172–79.

Page 11. Since then, our food environment has changed...: Boyd Swinburn, Gary Sacks, and Eric Ravussin, "Increased Food Energy Supply Is More Than Sufficient to Explain the US Epidemic of Obesity," *American Journal of Clinical Nutrition* 90 (December 2009): 1453–56, http://ajcn.nutrition.org/content/early/2009/10/14/ajcn.2009.28595.

Page 12. The number of calories available in the food supply...: "Food Availability (Per Capita) Data System, Overview," USDA/Economic Research Service Web site, last modified November 7, 2012, http://www.ers.usda.gov/data-products/food-availability-%28per-capita%29-data-system.aspx.

Page 12. Food companies not only had to compete for sales...: The "shareholder-value movement" is often attributed to a speech, "Growing Fast in a Slow-Growth Economy," given by Jack Welch in 1981. See Betty Morris, "The New Rules," *Fortune*, July 24, 2006, http://money.cnn.com/magazines/fortune/fortune_archive/2006/07/24/8381625/index.htm.

Page 13. And restaurants began serving foods...: T. A. Farley et al., "The Ubiquity of Energy-Dense Snack Foods: A National Multicity Study," *American Journal of Public Health* 100, no. 2 (February 2010): 306–11; see also L. R. Young and M. Nestle, "Reducing Portion Sizes to Prevent Obesity: A Call to Action," *American Journal of Preventive Medicine* 43, no. 5 (November 2012): 565–68, http://www.foodpolitics.com/wp-content/uploads/YoungPortions_AJPM_12.pdf.

CHAPTER 2

Page 20. Economists estimate that 22 percent...: A. Coleman-Jensen et al., "Household Food Security in the United States in 2011," *USDA/ERS Economic Research Report* No. ERR-141, September 2012, http://www.ers.usda.gov/publications/err-economic-research-report/err141.aspx. For current figures, see http://www.ers.usda.gov/topics/food-nutrition-assistance/food-security-in-the-us.aspx; see also "Poverty in the United States," National Poverty Center, http://www.npc.umich.edu/poverty/#5.

Page 21. Although the average benefit was only...: Center for the Study of the Presidency and Congress, *SNAP to Health: A Fresh Approach to Strengthening the Supplemental Nutrition Assistance Program* (Washington, DC, July 2012), http://www.thepresidency.org/storage/documents/CSPC_SNAP_Report.pdf. Updated figures for SNAP expenditures are at http://www.fns.usda.gov/pd/SNAPsummary.htm.

Page 22. Whether these can possibly meet the needs...: Janet Poppendieck, *Sweet Charity? Emergency Food and the End of Entitlement* (New York: Viking, 1998).

Page 26. The Food and Agriculture Organization of the United Nations...: Food and Agriculture Organization of the United Nations, "The State of Food Insecurity in the World, 2012," http://www.fao.org/docrep/016/i3027e/i3027e00.htm.

Page 31. The US government authorized large shipments...: "U.S. Aid Efforts in Libya," Voice of America (editorial), May 10, 2011, http://www.voanews.com/policy/editorials/US-Aid-Efforts-in-Libya--121603409.html.

Page 33. And does its nutritional quality...: "Food Aid," USDA Web site, http://www.fas.usda.gov/food-aid.asp; see also Mark E. Manyin and Mary Beth Nikitin, *Foreign Assistance to North Korea*, Congressional Research Service Report R40095, April 26, 2012, http://www.fas.org/sgp/crs/row/R40095.pdf.

CHAPTER 3

Page 37. Food is easily accessible, and today's society...: Much of this chapter is drawn from my book, *Why Calories Count* (Berkeley: University of California Press, 2012).

Page 39. Any level of overweight can raise the risk...: K. M. Flegal et al., "Association of All-Cause Mortality with Overweight and Obesity Using Standard Body Mass Index Categories: A Systematic Review and Meta-Analysis," *JAMA* 309, no. 1 (2013): 71–82.

Page 48. It views the food environment as a national...: J. Cawley and C. Meyerhoefer, "The Medical Care Costs of Obesity: An Instrumental Variables Approach," *Journal of Health Economics* 31, no. 1 (January 2012): 219–30; see also Mission Readiness, *Still Too Fat to Fight,* a follow-up report, September 2012, http://missionreadiness.s3.amazonaws.com/wp-content/uploads/Still-Too-Fat-To-Fight-Report.pdf.

CHAPTER 4

Page 52. As long as its purpose was to encourage eating...: Part I of my book *Food Politics* (Berkeley: University of California Press, 2013) reviews the history of dietary guidance in the United States and the development of food guide pyramids. The National Agricultural Library publishes historical food guides at http://fnic.nal.usda.gov/dietary-guidance/myplatefood-pyramid-resources.

Page 65. Although USDA economists argue about the meaning...: Fred Kuchler and Hayden Stewart, "Price Trends Are Similar for Fruits, Vegetables, and Snack Foods," USDA/ERS Economic Research Report No. ERR-55, March 2008, http://www.ers.usda.gov/publications/err-economic-research-report/err55.aspx.

Page 66. But research—much of it paid for by cereal companies...: Celeste A. Clark, *Cereal: The Complete Story,* Kellogg Company, 2010, http://www2.kelloggs.com/uploadedFiles/KelloggV9/Family/Carnegie_Compendium_FINAL.pdf. But see also Jennifer L. Harris et al., Cereal F.A.C.T.S.: Food Advertising to Children and Teens Score 2012, Yale Rudd Center, June 2012, http://www.cerealfacts.org/media/Cereal_FACTS_Report_2012_7.12.pdf.

CHAPTER 5

Page 69. Dietary recommendations apply to...: *Dietary Guidelines for Americans, 2010* is at http://health.gov/dietaryguidelines/2010.asp.

Page 73. Researchers who study children's food preferences...: S. L. Anzman, B. Y. Rollins, and L. L. Birch, "Parental Influence on Children's Early Eating Environments and Obesity Risk: Implications for Prevention," *International Journal of Obesity* 34, no. 7 (July 2010): 1116–24.

Page 75. Taste is critical, but research shows...: 100 Leading National Advertisers, *Advertising Age*, June 25, 2012, http://adage.com/article/datacenter-advertising-spending/100-leading-national-advertisers/234882/; see also T. N. Robinson et al., "Effects of Fast Food Branding on Young Children's Taste Preferences," *Archives of Pediatric and Adolescent Medicine* 161, no. 8 (2007): 792–97.

Page 78. Obesity is just as bad for the health...: "Childhood Obesity Facts," CDC Web site, http://www.cdc.gov/healthyyouth/obesity/facts.htm.

Page 78. Pediatricians advise parents who are concerned...: F. J. Zimmerman and J. F. Bell, "Associations of Television Content Type and Obesity in Children," *American Journal of Public Health* 100, no. 2 (February 2010): 334–40.

Page 79. They also make large donations...: Coca-Cola, "The Coca-Cola Foundation Awards $17.9 Million to 83 Organizations Worldwide during Fourth Quarter," press release, December 6, 2011, http://www.thecoca-colacompany.com/dynamic/press_center/2011/12/the-coca-cola-foundation-4th-quarter-grants.html.

Page 84. They particularly objected to the use of ammonia...: Bettina Elias Siegel, "How My 'Pink Slime' Petition Took Off," *Guardian*, April 6, 2012, http://www.guardian.co.uk/commentisfree/cifamerica/2012/apr/06/pink-slime-rebellion-beef.

Page 86. In 2011, the USDA school breakfast program served...: Information about the USDA's meal programs are at the National School Lunch Program page, http://www.fns.usda.gov/cnd/Lunch, and the School Breakfast Program page, http://www.fns.usda.gov/cnd/Breakfast/Default.htm.

Page 87. Schools across the country have transformed...: Janet Poppendieck, *Free for All: Fixing School Food in America* (Berkeley: University of California Press, 2010).

Page 88. The agency also set nutrient-based standards...: "Nutrition Standards for School Meals," January 26, 2012, USDA Web site, http://www.fns.usda.gov/cnd/governance/legislation/nutritionstandards.htm.

CHAPTER 6

Page 95. They cite other ways to reduce heart disease risk...: *Dietary Guidelines for Americans, 2010*, http://www.health.gov/dietaryguidelines/2010.asp.

Page 96. Americans bought more than $11 billion worth...: "Dietary Supplement Fact Sheet: Multivitamin/Mineral Supplements," NIH Office of Dietary Supplements Web site, last reviewed January 7, 2013, http://ods.od.nih.gov/factsheets/MVMS-HealthProfessional.

Page 98. Hundreds of firms manufacture pet food products...: "Industry Statistics & Trends," American Pet Products Association Web site, http://www.americanpetproducts.org/press_industrytrends.asp.

Page 99. Whether revolting to us or not...: Marion Nestle, *Feed Your Pet Right: The Authoritative Guide to Feeding Your Dog and Cat* (New York: Free Press, 2010).

Page 99. If this could happen to dogs and cats...: Marion Nestle, *Pet Food Politics: The Chihuahua in the Coal Mine* (Berkeley: University of California Press, 2008).

Page 100. The most commonly transferred characteristics...: Marion Nestle, *Safe Food: The Politics of Food Safety* (Berkeley: University of California Press, 2010), Introduction and Part II, Chapters 5–8.

Page 105. Since 1994, the FDA has approved genetically...: "Completed Consultations on Bioengineered Foods," FDA Web site, last updated August 31, 2012, http://www.accessdata.fda.gov/scripts/fcn/fcnNavigation.cfm?rpt=bioListing.

Page 108. The FDA says these are safe for human...: "Animal Cloning," FDA Web site, last updated April 26, 2010, http://www.fda.gov/AnimalVeterinary/SafetyHealth/AnimalCloning/default.htm.

CHAPTER 7

Page 111. Indeed, as Secretary of Health and Human Services...: William Branigin, Mike Allen, and John Mintz, "Tommy Thompson Resigns from HHS," *Washington Post*, December 3, 2004, http://www.washingtonpost.com/wp-dyn/articles/A31377-2004Dec3.html. For a more detailed discussion of food safety issues, see my book, *Safe Food*, Part I, chapters 1–4.

Page 113. The FDA did not propose rules to implement...: "The New Food Safety Modernization Act (FSMA)," FDA Web site, last updated January 8, 2013, http://www.fda.gov/food/foodsafety/fsma/default.htm.

Page 114. The CDC estimated that foodborne microbial illnesses…: "Estimates of Foodborne Illness in the United States," CDC Web site, last updated January 28, 2013, http://www.cdc.gov/foodborneburden/.

Page 119. Despite hazardous production standards…: The FDA page on the peanut butter recall is http://www.fda.gov/Safety/Recalls/MajorProductRecalls/Peanut/default.htm; see also "Investigation Update: Outbreak of *Salmonella* Typhimurium Infections, 2008–2009," CDC Web site, April 29, 2009, www.cdc.gov/salmonella/typhimurium/update.html. The legalities of this incident and the one involving eggs (see the next note) are reviewed by Bill Marler, an attorney who represents victims of food poisonings. See Bill Marler, "Will the Jensen Brothers, DeCoster and Parnell Ever Meet in the Big House?" *Marler Blog*, June 10, 2012, http://www.marlerblog.com/lawyer-oped/will-the-jensen-brothers-decoster-and-parnell-ever-meet-in-the-big-house/#.UPsYkXdXnj5.

Page 120. After-the-fact investigations revealed a long history…: "Investigation Update: Multistate Outbreak of Human *Salmonella* Enteritidis Infections Associated with Shell Eggs," CDC Web site, December 2, 2010, http://www.cdc.gov/salmonella/enteritidis; see also "Recall of Shell Eggs," FDA Web site, October 18, 2010, http://www.fda.gov/Safety/Recalls/MajorProductRecalls/ucm223522.htm#483.

Page 121. These kill bacteria with reasonable…: "Food Irradiation," EPA Web site, last updated June 27, 2012, http://www.epa.gov/rpdweb00/sources/food_irrad.html.

Page 123. Consumers cannot easily avoid these chemicals…: Environmental Working Group, "EWG's 2012 Shoppers' Guide to Pesticides in Produce," June 19, 2012, http://www.ewg.org/foodnews.

Page 124. The FDA says that BPA is safe…: "Bisphenol A (BPA) Information for Parents," HHS Web site, n.d., http://www.hhs.gov/safety/bpa; see also "Bisphenol A (BPA)," FDA Web site, last updated July 26, 2012, http://www.fda.gov/food/foodingredientspackaging/ucm166145.htm.

Page 124. Pregnant women must take care to avoid…: "What You Need to Know about Mercury in Fish and Shellfish," March 2004, FDA Web site, http://www.fda.gov/food/foodsafety/product-specificinformation/seafood/foodbornepathogenscontaminants/methylmercury/ucm115662.htm.

Page 127. The agency trained 40 inspectors to sniff out…: Associated Press, "Oil Spill Seafood Testers Sniff Out Tainted Fish, Shrimp, Oysters at Pascagoula Lab (with video)," June 7, 2010, http://blog.gulflive.com/mississippi-press-news/2010/06/oil_spill_seafood_testers_snif.html.

Page 128. But such an answer is hardly…: "Radiation Safety," FDA Web site, last updated June 21, 2012, http://www.fda.gov/newsevents/publichealthfocus/ucm247403.htm.

Page 129. By the early 2000s, mad cow…: Nestle, *Safe Food*, 250–55.

Page 131. Since testing began, officials have identified…: "BSE (Bovine Spongiform Encephalopathy, or Mad Cow Disease)," CDC Web site, September 14, 2012, http://www.cdc.gov/ncidod/dvrd/bse.

Page 132. Because downer cows are at high risk…: "Questions and Answers Hallmark/Westland Beef Packing Co," USDA Web site, March 7, 2008, http://www.usda.gov/wps/portal/usda/usdahome?contentid=2008/02/0048.xml&contentidonly=true.

CHAPTER 8

Page 135. These foods are made with inexpensive…: Many of the issues mentioned in this section are discussed and referenced in my book, *What to Eat* (New York: North Point Press, 2006). Resources on food and beverage marketing are available from the Food Marketing Workgroup, http://www.foodmarketing.org.

Page 138. Much research has gone into explaining…: P. Chandon and B. Wansink, "Does Food Marketing Need to Make Us Fat? A Review and Solutions," *Nutrition Reviews* 70, no. 10 (October 2012): 571–93.

Page 141. The FDA dealt with these requirements…: "How to Understand and Use the Nutrition Facts Label," FDA Web site, last updated February 15, 2012, http://www.fda.gov/Food/ResourcesForYou/Consumers/NFLPM/ucm274593.htm.

Page 144. But these products seem anything but…: The Mayo Clinic reviews the current status of artificial sweeteners in "Artificial Sweeteners and Other Sugar Substitutes," at its Web site, http://www.mayoclinic.com/health/artificial-sweeteners/MY00073.

Page 145. People take in excessive calories…: "100 Leading National Advertisers," *Advertising Age*, June 20, 2010, http://adage.com/article/datacenter-advertising-spending/100-leading-national-advertisers/144208/; see also B. Wansink and P. Chandon, "Can 'Low-Fat' Nutrition Labels Lead to Obesity?" *Journal of Marketing Research* 43, no. 4 (November 2006): 605–17; see also Brian Wansink, *Mindless Eating: Why We Eat More Than We Think* (New York: Bantam, 2006): 1.

Page 146. Because so many companies invented...: For information about the FDA's efforts to regulate front-of-package labeling standards, see Institute of Medicine, *Front-of-Package Nutrition Rating Systems and Symbols: Promoting Healthier Choices* (Washington, DC: National Academies Press, 2012), http://www.iom.edu/Reports/2011/Front-of-Package-Nutrition-Rating-Systems-and-Symbols-Promoting-Healthier-Choices.aspx.

CHAPTER 9

Page 151. Federal policies support the current food environment...: For an analysis of the effects of farm subsidies on health, see Heather Schoonover and Mark Muller, *Food without Thought: How U.S. Farm Policy Contributes to Obesity* (Minneapolis: Institute for Agriculture and Trade Policy, 2006), http://www.iatp.org/files/421_2_80627.pdf.

Page 151. And because removing them from the food supply...: D. Mozaffarian et al., "Trans Fatty Acids and Cardiovascular Disease," *New England Journal of Medicine* 354 (2006): 1601–13.

Page 152. Restaurant owners like using partially hydrogenated...: The label can indicate 0 gram trans fat as long as the amount is less than 0.5 gram per serving. For FDA labeling information, see "Labeling & Nutrition: Food Labeling and Nutrition Overview," http://www.fda.gov/food/labelingnutrition/default.htm.

Page 153. A year later, the board voted to restrict...: The New York City trans fat ban is at www.nyc.gov/html/doh/downloads/pdf/public/notice-adoption-hc-art81-08.pdf.

Page 154. But studies show that restaurants are now using...: S. Y. Angell et al., "Change in Trans Fatty Acid Content of Fast-Food Purchases Associated with New York City's Restaurant Regulation: A Pre-Post Study," *Annals of Internal Medicine* 157, no. 2 (2012): 81–86; see also Alice H. Lichtenstein, "New York City Trans Fat Ban: Improving the Default Option When Purchasing Foods Prepared Outside of the Home," *Annals of Internal Medicine* 157, no. 2 (2012): 144–5, http://annals.org/article.aspx?articleid=1216555.

Page 156. An investigative report suggested that the White House...: The FDA's original guidance, now replaced, is: "WITHDRAWN–Draft Guidance for Industry: Questions and Answers Regarding Implementation of the Menu Labeling Provisions of Section 4205 of the Patient Protection and Affordable Care Act of 2010," August 2010, http://www.fda.gov/Food/GuidanceComplianceRegulatoryInformation/GuidanceDocuments/FoodLabelingNutrition/ucm223266.htm. For current FDA menu labeling documents, see "New Menu and Vending Machines Labeling Requirements," http://www.fda.gov/food/labelingnutrition/ucm217762.htm. See also Gardiner Harris, "White House and the F.D.A. Often at Odds," *New York Times*, April 2, 2012, http://www.nytimes.com/2012/04/03/health/policy/white-house-and-fda-at-odds-on-regulatory-issues.html?_r=4&pagewanted=1&hp.

Page 158. All failed as a result of extensive lobbying...: Duane D. Stanford, "Anti-Obesity Soda Tax Fails as Lobbyists Spend Millions: Retail," *Business Week*, March 13, 2012, www.businessweek.com/news/2012-03-13/anti-obesity-soda-tax-fails-as-lobbyists-spend-millions-retail#p1; see also Kate Sheppard, "Beverage Industry Group Bankrolls Soda Tax Opposition," *Mother Jones*, July 25, 2012, www.motherjones.com/environment/2012/07/meet-beverage-industry-group-bankrolls-soda-tax-opposition.

Page 159. Health department studies indicated that more than...: Michael M. Grynbaum, "New York Plans to Ban Sale of Big Sizes of Sugary Drinks," *New York Times*, May 30, 2012, www.nytimes.com/2012/05/31/nyregion/bloomberg-plans-a-ban-on-large-sugared-drinks.html?_r=3. For relevant documents, see New York City Department of Health and Mental Hygiene—Nutrition and Physical Activity, "Sugary Drinks," http://www.nyc.gov/html/doh/html/living/cdp_pan_pop.shtml.

Page 161. In doing so, the soda industry was positioning itself...: Michael M. Grynbaum, "Fighting Ban on Big Sodas with Appeals to Patriotism," *New York Times*, July 23, 2012, http://cityroom.blogs.nytimes.com/2012/07/23/a-rally-for-sweet-drink-rights-comes-with-soaked-in-patriotism.

CHAPTER 10

Page 166. Industrial agriculture is estimated to account...: Lappé, *Diet for a Hot Planet* (New York, Bloomsbury USA, 2010).

Page 172. In the United States, the USDA sets standards...: "National Organic Program," USDA Web site, last modified November 28, 2012, http://www.ams.usda.gov/AMSv1.0/nop.

Page 174. Organic foods and beverages accounted for...: Organic Trade Association, "Consumer-Driven U.S. Organic Market Surpasses $31 Billion in 2011," press release, April 23, 2012, http://www.organicnewsroom.com/2012/04/us_consumerdriven_organic_mark.html. The association's industry statistics are at http://www.ota.com/organic/mt/business.html.

The work of these 40 cartoonists—and several others—may be searched online at CartoonistGroup.com.

NICK ANDERSON is the editorial cartoonist at the *Houston Chronicle* and the winner of the 2005 Pulitzer Prize. His cartoons are syndicated by the *Washington Post* Writers Group. He began his career at the *Louisville Courier-Journal* after graduating from Ohio State University. He is the father of Colton and Travis, whose names are hidden in his cartoons, which can be found online at http://blog.chron.com/nickanderson.

DARRIN BELL started to draw as a child in South Los Angeles and developed the concept for "Candorville," syndicated by the *Washington Post* Writers Group, while attending the University of California at Berkeley, where he now lives. When "Candorville" began syndication in 2003, it was one of the few strips distributed in both Spanish and English in the United States. Bell also collaborates with Theron Heir on the comic strip "Rudy Park." "Candorville" is online at www.candorville.com.

CLAY BENNETT is the editorial cartoonist for the *Chattanooga Times Free Press*. His work is syndicated by the *Washington Post* Writers Group. Nominated for the Pulitzer more often than any cartoonist alive today (winning the prize in 2002), Bennett has won every major editorial cartoon award. He lives in Chattanooga with his wife, Cindy Procious, and their children, Matt, Ben, and Sarah. His work can be found at www.timesfreepress.com/news/opinion/cartoons/.

LISA BENSON is a freelance artist, graphic designer, and cartoonist who has drawn editorial cartoons for the *Victor Valley (California) Daily Press* since 1992. They are syndicated by the *Washington Post* Writers Group. Her work has been recognized with numerous awards, and she lives in Apple Valley with her husband, Gregory, and their four children. See Benson's cartoons online at www.vvdailypress.com/sections/opinion.

CHIP BOK's cartoons are syndicated by Creators Syndicate, and they appear regularly in newspapers and magazines throughout the United States. Among his many awards are Editorial Cartoonist of the Year given by *The Week* magazine (2007) and Top 10 Political Cartoons given by *Time* (2008). Bok has published two cartoon compilations and also coauthored a children's book, *The Great White House Breakout*, with Helen

Thomas. Bok lives in Akron, Ohio, with his wife, Deborah, and their children. Visit www.bokbluster.com to see his cartoons.

JIM BORGMAN's cartooning career has included work in both editorial cartoons and comic strips. He currently collaborates with Jerry Scott on the strip "Zits," which was launched in 1997 and is syndicated by King Features. Borgman retired from his job as the editorial cartoonist at the *Cincinnati Enquirer* in 2008. Borgman has won the Pulitzer Prize for Editorial Cartoons (1991), the Reuben Award for Best Editorial Cartoons (an unprecedented five times in 1986, 1987, 1988, 1994, and 2006), and the Reuben Award for Best Newspaper Comic Strip (1998 and 1999). Borgman and his wife, Suzanne, live in Cincinnati with their five children. "Zits" is located online at www.zitscomics.com.

DAVE COVERLY is the creator of "Speed Bump," syndicated by Creators Syndicate, and the winner of the 2008 Reuben Award for Outstanding Cartoonist of the Year. He works in Ann Arbor, Michigan, with inspiration from his close friend, Cuppa Joe. He lives with his wife, Chris, and their daughters, Alayna and Simone. His work can be found at www.speedbump.com.

BRIAN CRANE creates his comic strip "Pickles" in Reno, Nevada, where he lives with his wife, Diana. They have raised seven children and multiple grandchildren. "Pickles" is set in Crane's hometown of Sparks, Nevada, and was introduced to newspaper readers in 1990. It is syndicated by the *Washington Post* Writers Group. Also available in several collections, "Pickles" has received multiple awards, including the Reuben Award for Best Comic Strip in 2001.

JEFF DANZIGER's editorial cartoons are seen worldwide and distributed by the CWS/*New York Times* Syndicate. The recipient of the Herblock Prize and the Thomas Nast (Landau) Prize for his work and the Bronze Star and the Air Medal for his service in Vietnam, he lives in New York City. He has published eleven books of cartoons and one novel. His work can be found at www.danzigercartoons.com.

JOHN DEERING, the editorial cartoonist at the *Arkansas Democrat-Gazette* and the creator of the comic strip "Strange Brew," has cartooned since he was three years old. After studying commercial and fine art, Deering began his career in advertising. He became the paper's editorial cartoonist in 1988, and "Strange Brew" followed in 1998. His cartoons have won multiple awards and are syndicated by Creators Syndicate. They may be found online at www.arkansasonline.com/staff/john-deering.

LIZA DONNELLY is a staff cartoonist at the *New Yorker*. She is also a public speaker and has spoken about cartooning at TED conferences, the United Nations, and the *New Yorker* Festival. Her many books include *Funny Ladies: The New Yorker's Greatest Women Cartoonists and Their Cartoons,* and she has been the driving force behind several well-regarded cartoon collections. As an editor, Donnelly conceived of World Ink. She also is a charter member of Cartooning for Peace. Donnelly lives in New York with her husband, *New Yorker* cartoonist Michael Maslin. See her cartoons at www.lizadonnelly.com.

GREG EVANS, the creator of the comic strip "Luann," received the 2003 Reuben Award for Outstanding Cartoonist of the Year. Evans developed the idea for "Luann" while working as a graphic artist and promotion manager for a television station and freelancing as a magazine cartoonist. Launched in 1985 and syndicated by Universal UClick, "Luann" has been compiled into several books as well as a series of pamphlets on important health topics for adolescents. It can be found online at www.luannsroom.com.

ALEX HALLATT grew up in England, lived briefly in the United States, emigrated to New Zealand, and now lives in Victoria, Australia. Her comic strip, "Arctic Circle," evolved from a strip she started while at the University of Kent. First published in 2005 as "Polar Circle" in Australia, it is now syndicated by King Features and can be found at www.arcticcirclecartoons.com.

JOHN HAMBROCK, the creator of the strip "The Brilliant Mind of Edison Lee," enjoys a successful career as both a graphic designer and cartoonist (foreshadowed by his being voted the Most Artistic Male as a high school senior). His wife, Anne, has been a driving force in his cartooning career and also helps with the coloring of the strip, which is syndicated by King Features and can be found at www.edisonlee.net.

LEE JUDGE is the editorial cartoonist at the *Kansas City Star*. He has the unusual distinction of also being a sports blogger. During baseball season, Judge blogs about the Kansas City Royals for the paper. He began his career at the *Sacramento Union*, moved to the *San Diego Union-Tribune*, and arrived in Kansas City in 1981. His cartoons are syndicated by King Features and can be found at www.kansascity.com/opinion/lee_judge.

STEVE KELLEY is an editorial cartoonist and cocreator of the comic strip "Dustin." Kelley began drawing cartoons in college for the *Daily Dartmouth* and the *Dartmouth Review*. In 1981, he went to work at the *San Diego Union-Tribune* and was the editorial cartoonist at the *New Orleans Times-Picayune* from 2001 to 2012. His editorial cartoons are syndicated by Creators Syndicate. "Dustin," a collaboration with Jeff Parker that launched in 2010, was awarded the Reuben Award for Best Newspaper Comic Strip its first year. It is syndicated by King Features.

RICK KIRKMAN says that he "was born a poor cartoonist in a log cabin drawn in poor perspective." His path to creating "Baby Blues" (with Jerry Scott) included work in advertising, freelance design, and drawing cartoons for magazines. First syndicated in 1990, "Baby Blues," syndicated by King Features, received the Reuben Award for Best Newspaper Comic Strip in 1995. In 2000, a successful prime-time animated show based on the comic strip was launched on The WB. Kirkman lives in Arizona with his wife and two children. The strip can be found at www.babyblues.com.

MIKE LUCKOVICH is a two-time winner of the Pulitzer Prize for Editorial Cartoons (1995 and 2006) and was also granted the Reuben Award for Outstanding Cartoonist of the Year (2006). His work appears in the *Atlanta Journal-Constitution* as well as many leading newspapers and magazines. Luckovich and his wife, Margo, have three children. Syndicated by Creators Syndicate, his cartoons can be found at www.blogs.ajc.com/mike-luckovich.

REX MAY, a gag cartoonist who frequently signs his cartoons as "Baloo," is a retired postal worker who now devotes himself full-time to writing and drawing. In the mid-1970s he wrote for *National Lampoon* and started gag writing for a number of syndicated columnists and cartoonists. He also draws his own cartoons, which have appeared in *Reader's Digest*, the *Wall Street Journal*, the *National Review,* and other publications. He lives with his wife, Jean, and their children, Freda, Tyr, and Bjorn. His work can be found at www.baloocartoons.com.

KIERAN MEEHAN, the creator of "Pros and Cons," describes himself as a "British Isles mongrel." He worked in the advertising and design fields for 20 years while he studied art and refined his skills as a cartoonist. Early strips such "Private Eye" and "Punch" led to his cartoons being included in "The New Breed" (King Features) and ultimately to "Pros and Cons," also syndicated by King Features. His work can be found at www.meehancartoons.com.

JEFF PARKER collaborates with Steve Kelley to create the comic strip "Dustin." He is also the editorial cartoonist at *Florida Today*. Parker and Kelley launched "Dustin" in 2010, when it was awarded the Reuben Award for Best Newspaper Comic Strip. When not working on "Dustin" and his editorial cartoons, Parker also assists Mike Peters with his comic strip "Mother Goose and Grimm." He works from his home studio. His wife, Pat, considers him to be her only child.

MIKE PETERS' favorite expression is "What a hoot!" This sums up his outlook on his life and his work, which are inexorably entwined. The creator of "Mother Goose and Grimm," he is also a Pulitzer Prize–winning editorial cartoonist whose work has been syndicated since 1971. "Mother Goose and Grimm" was born in 1984 with the help of Marian, his wife, best friend, and business partner of 40 years. Both his comic strip and editorial cartoons are syndicated by King Features and may be seen online at www.grimmy.com.

JOEL PETT, winner of the 2000 Pulitzer Prize for Editorial Cartoons, has been the editorial cartoonist at the *Lexington Herald-Leader* since 1984. Having observed life in more than 25 countries—from his boyhood home in Nigeria, down the Amazon, Red Square, Tiananmen Square, and beyond—Pett sums up his philosophy simply: "Hello, God? Listen, we could use some help down here." His cartoons are distributed by CWS/*New York Times* Syndicate and are online at www.kentucky.com/joel-pett.

RINA PICCOLO's strip "Tina's Groove" and her panel cartoons appear in numerous magazines, including the *New Yorker* and *Parade* magazine. Also a contributor to "Six Chix," she began her professional career in 1989 with her first published cartoon, and she's been happily chained to the drawing board ever since. Piccolo lives in Toronto, where she was born and raised. "Tina's Groove" is syndicated by King Features, and all of her work may be seen online at www.rinapiccolo.com.

DAN PIRARO was the 2009 winner of the Reuben Award for Outstanding Cartoonist of the Year. His strip "Bizarro," syndicated by King Features, won the Reuben Award for Best Newspaper Comic Strip in 2000, 2001, and 2002. Piraro's cartoons have been reprinted in 16 book collections, and he has written three books of prose. In 2006, the HSUS recognized Piraro's animal rights activism by awarding him its highest honor, the Genesis Award for Ongoing Commitment. Piraro was born and raised in the dead center of the United States; his work can be found at www.bizarro.com.

DWANE POWELL spent the majority of his career—from 1975 to 2009—as the editorial cartoonist at the *Raleigh News & Observer*. Previously, he had been a cartoonist at the *San Antonio Light*. While still in college at the University of Arkansas at Monticello, his first cartoons were published in the *Arkansas Gazette*, and his career began at the *Hot Springs Sentinel Record*. Powell lives in Raleigh with his wife, Jan. They have a daughter and a grandchild. His work is syndicated by Creators Syndicate.

HILARY PRICE, the creator of the comic strip "Rhymes with Orange," syndicated by King Features, became the youngest female syndicated cartoonist in the country when her strip launched in 1995. "Rhymes with Orange" received the 2007 Reuben Award for Best Cartoon Panel. A Stanford graduate, Price's early career included work as an advertising copywriter and a brief stint as a journalist. She now lives back in her home state of Massachusetts with her partner, Kerry, and their geriatric pets. Her work can be found at www.rhymeswithorange.com.

JERRY SCOTT is the cocreator of two comic strips, "Baby Blues" and "Zits," both syndicated by King Features. They have been awarded the Reuben Award for Best Newspaper Comic Strip, and Scott also received the Reuben Award for Outstanding Cartoonist of the Year in 2001. Scott entered the newspaper business via predawn bike rides as a paperboy in his hometown of South Bend, Indiana, when he could be the first person in his neighborhood to read the comics. He lives in California with his wife, Kim, and their two daughters. His work can be found at www.babyblues.com and www.zitscomics.com.

MIKE SMITH has drawn editorial cartoons for more than 20 years at the *Las Vegas Sun,* which ran his first cartoon while he was still in college. Smith also draws a weekly cartoon for *USA Today* and creates "StockcarToon," a weekly NASCAR strip. His work has appeared in the *Los Angeles Times*, the *Washington Post*, *Time* magazine, and numerous other publications. His cartoons are syndicated by King Features and can be found at www.lasvegassun.com/news/opinion/smiths-world.

JEN SORENSEN's comics and illustrations appear in alternative newsweeklies and magazines and on Web sites such as *Daily Kos*. She also has created cartoons specifically for NPR.org and KaiserHealthNews.org. Her work has won seven awards from the Association of Alternative Newsweeklies, including first place in 2012. Also named as a 2012 Herblock Prize finalist, she lives in Austin, Texas, with her husband and a small "Toto-like canine unit." Sorensen self-syndicates her cartoons, which can be seen at www.jensorensen.com.

BOB STAAKE is a cartoonist, illustrator, designer, and author. His illustrations have appeared in countless publications and on the cover of the *New Yorker* several times, including those selected by *AdAge* as among the best magazine covers of 2008, 2010, and 2012. He is the author and illustrator of more than 50 children's books. A native of Torrance, California, Staake and his wife, Paulette, live on Cape Cod with their son, Ryan. His work can be found at www.bobstaake.com.

JAY STEPHENS, a cocreator of "Oh, Brother!", syndicated by King Features, is an Emmy-award–winning Canadian cartoonist and creator of the children's television programs

Tutenstein and *The Secret Saturdays*. His work as a cartoonist includes alternative comics such as *The Land of Nod*, *Atomic City Tales,* as well as his contributions to licensed comics such as *Batman* and *Felix the Cat*. Stephens lives in Guelph, Ontario, and his work can be found at www.ohbrothercomics.com.

ANN TELNAES took the unusual path of beginning her career in national syndication rather than as a staff cartoonist. Now as staff jobs disappear, Telnaes is the country's only animated editorial cartoonist at the *Washington Post*. Only the second woman to receive the Pulitzer Prize for Editorial Cartoons (2001), she also worked with The Cartoonist Group in 2012 to produce the first-ever editorial cartoon app, "POTUS Pick." Her print cartoons are available from The Cartoonist Group, and her Web site is www.anntelnaes.com.

BOB AND TOM THAVES are the father-son duo responsible for "Frank and Ernest." Bob, the father, created the strip, and Tom began to work on it in the late 1990s. Upon Bob's death in 2006, Tom assumed full responsibility for the comic strip and now collaborates with a team to create it. "Frank and Ernest" has received the Reuben Award for being the Best Cartoon Panel three times and is syndicated by Universal UClick. When not producing cartoons, Tom Thaves is more than likely thinking about them as he surfs in the waters off San Diego, where he lives. See "Frank and Ernest" online at www.frankandernest.com.

BRUCE TINSLEY, creator of "Mallard Fillmore," was born in Louisville, Kentucky, and has been a reporter, editorial writer, and copy editor for newspapers in Kentucky, Virginia, and Washington, DC. Tinsley was a Reader's Digest Fellow at Indiana University's graduate school of journalism and acknowledges that the main character in his comic strip is based wholly on himself.

MIKE TWOHY is the cartoonist of "That's Life." His comic strip fulfills an ambition that began with his first submission to syndicates at age 11—"I just remember being delighted that the rejection letters addressed me as Mr. Twohy"—and he honed his skill as a cartoonist by freelancing for various markets. He sold his first cartoon to the *New Yorker* in 1980, which has published his cartoons regularly since. "That's Life" is available from The Cartoonist Group.

GARY VARVEL is the editorial cartoonist for the *Indianapolis Star*. Varvel studied visual communication at Indiana University and began his career at the paper as an artist. Varvel spends his mornings as a part-time art teacher for Bethesda Christian School High School in Brownsburg, Indiana. His cartoons are syndicated by Creators and may be seen online at www.townhall.com/political-cartoons/garyvarvel

BOB WEBER, JR., is a cocreator of "Oh, Brother!", which was distributed to newspapers by King Features. He also created "Skylock Fox and Comics for Kids." Weber began to cartoon in college, following in the footsteps of his father, who created the comic strip "Moose and Molly." His work can be found at www. ohbrothercomics.com.

SIGNE WILKINSON is an editorial cartoonist for the *Philadelphia Daily News* and the creator of the comic strip "Family Tree." Wilkinson was the first woman to receive the Pulitzer Prize for Editorial Cartoons in 1992, and her award-winning work has been syndicated by the *Washington Post* Writers Group. Wilkinson and her husband live in Philadelphia with two birds, five goldfish, and a dog named Ginger. Her Web site is www.signetoons.com.

MATT WUERKER is a political cartoonist, founding staff member at *Politico*, and winner of the 2012 Pulitzer Prize for Editorial Cartoons. His career has included work in clay animation with Will Vinton; illustrating the work of Dr. Laurence Peter; and artwork on music videos for artists including Michael Jackson, Joni Mitchell, Paul Simon, and others. Wuerker lives with his wife, Sarah, and their son, Ryan, in Washington, DC. His cartoons may be seen online at www. politico.com/wuerker/.

CARTOON CREDITS

John Deering Editorial Cartoons:
Published originally in the *Arkansas Democrat-Gazette*.
p. 109 – January 17, 2008
p. 161 – June 14, 2012

Liza Donnelly Panel Cartoons:
Published originally at LizaDonnelly.com.
p. 74 – May 27, 2011
p. 179 – April 19, 2011

Dustin by Steve Kelley and Jeff Parker: Distributed to newspapers by King Features Syndicate.
p. 37 – July 27, 2011
p. 41 – July 28, 2011
p. 146 – August 13, 2011

Family Tree by Signe Wilkinson:
Distributed to newspapers by United Media/Universal Press.
p. 46 – September 8, 2010
p. 56 – July 17, 2011
p. 59 – April 8, 2009
p. 85 – September 24, 2010
p. 166 – January 12, 2009
p. 169 – May 13, 2009
p. 172 – September 23, 2010
p. 174 – July 15, 2009
p. 174 – December 5, 2010
p. 175 – May 24, 2010
p. 180 – December 18, 2008
p. 180 – December 19, 2008

Frank and Ernest by Bob and Tom Thaves: Distributed to newspapers by United Media/Universal Press.
p. xvi – April 20, 1978
p. xvii – June 21, 2008
p. 2 – June 7, 2006
p. 5 – May 16, 2004
p. 15 – October 11, 1994
p. 76 – July 23, 2008
p. 82 – December 7, 2006
p. 86 – September 6, 2011
p. 97 – October 23, 1998
p. 107 – April 6, 2012
p. 112 – May 31, 2006
p. 133 – April 9, 2001
p. 136 – March 16, 2003
p. 138 – April 10, 2003
p. 139 – June 8, 2007

p. 141 – April 28, 1994
p. 144 – February 7, 2005
p. 181 – August 25, 2004

Lee Judge Editorial Cartoons:
Published originally in the *Kansas City Star*.
p. 3 – August 22, 2010
p. 36 – October 26, 2011
p. 49 – July 24, 2011
p. 55 – September 28, 2010
p. 96 – October 13, 2011
p. 106 – September 24, 2010
p. 158 – March 14, 2010
p. 160 – June 13, 2012

Steve Kelley Editorial Cartoons:
Unless otherwise noted, published originally in the *Times–Picayune* New Orleans.
p. xiii – February 27, 2009
p. xiv – January 31, 2005
p. xvii – August 15, 2010
p. xix – June 22, 2009
p. 12 – August 23, 2012
p. 14 – October 26, 2004
p. 45 – January 1, 1999*
*Published originally in the *San Diego Union-Tribune*.
p. 47 – March 11, 2004
p. 54 – April 29, 2005
p. 57 – July 11, 2012
p. 62 – March 13, 2011
p. 75 – April 5, 2004
p. 82 – September 15, 2006
p. 96 – July 27, 2007
p. 120 – August 25, 2010
p. 123 – May 3, 2007
p. 127 – August 3, 2010
p. 131 – January 2, 2004
p. 133 – December 29, 2003
p. 152 – November 1, 2006
p. 153 – March 1, 2007
p. 154 – September 29, 2006
p. 157 – May 15, 2009
p. 162 – May 24, 2004
p. 162 – June 18, 2007

Luann by Greg Evans: Distributed to newspapers by United Media/Universal Press.
p. 13 – February 11, 2009

Mike Luckovich Editorial Cartoons:
Published originally in the *Atlanta Journal–Constitution*.
p. 58 – March 14, 2012
p. 119 – February 17, 2009
p. 120 – January 27, 2009
p. 161 – September 14, 2012

Mallard Fillmore by Bruce Tinsley:
Distributed to newspapers by King Features Syndicate.
p. 27 – May 12, 2011
p. 169 – October 18, 2011
p. 170 – May 29, 2012

Rex May Panel Cartoons: Published originally at Baloocartoons.com.
p. 58 – February 18, 2009
p. 66 – August 19, 2008
p. 105 – June 16, 2007
p. 137 – June 3, 2008

Mother Goose and Grimm by Mike Peters: Distributed to newspapers by King Features Syndicate.
p. 15 – May 13, 2008
p. 98 – June 29, 2002
p. 125 – February 14, 2006
p. 156 – August 5, 2011
p. 156 – May 25, 2012
p. 178 – September 17, 2007

Oh, Brother! by Jay Stephens and Bob Weber, Jr.: Distributed to newspapers by King Features Syndicate.
p. 67 – March 5, 2011
p. 71 – June 29, 2011

Mike Peters Editorial Cartoons:
Published originally in the *Dayton Daily News*.
Cover and p. x – November 17, 2011
p. 42 – March 18, 2004
p. 65 – May 23, 2004
p. 107 – November 7, 2003
p. 128 – March 16, 2011

Joel Pett Editorial Cartoons: Unless otherwise noted, published originally in the *Lexington Herald-Leader*.
p. 26 – August 6, 2008
p. 30 – July 29, 2008

p. 31 – June 14, 2011
p. 32 – March 25, 2011
p. 86 – March 20, 2002
p. 88 – February 12, 2003
p. 105 – March 28, 2001
p. 122 – March 10, 2010

Rina Piccolo Panel Cartoons:
Published originally at Rinapiccolo.com.
p. 97 – September 30, 2009

Pickles by Brian Crane: Distributed
to newspapers by the *Washington Post*
Writers Group.
p. 72 – February 9, 2012
p. 72 – June 10, 2008
p. 72 – April 6, 2012

Dwane Powell Editorial Cartoons:
Published originally in the *Raleigh News
and Observer*.
p. 88 – April 7, 2006
p. 113 – March 9, 2009
p. 117 – May 10, 2007
p. 125 – April 26, 2006

Pros and Cons by Kieran Meehan:
Distributed to newspapers by King
Features Syndicate.
p. 60 – January 25, 2009

**Rhymes with Orange by Hilary
Price:** Distributed to newspapers by
King Features Syndicate.
p. 39 – September 20, 2009
p. 42 – September 16, 2010
p. 61 – March 3, 2012
p. 63 – August 7, 2009
p. 70 – March 28, 2012
p. 136 – January 4, 2012
p. 142 – March 28, 2011
p. 143 – November 12, 2009
p. 150 – April 23, 2012
p. 170 – August 16, 2012

Mike Smith Editorial Cartoons:
Published originally in the *Las Vegas
Sun*.
p. 44 – February 4, 2012

Jen Sorensen Editorial Cartoons:
Published originally at Jensorensen.com.

p. 80 – August 13, 2012
p. 84 – June 1, 2012
p. 89 – November 21, 2011
p. 140 – November 1, 2010
p. 163 – April 4, 2011

Speed Bump by Dave Coverly:
Distributed to newspapers by Creators
Syndicate.
p. 7 – April 23, 2004
p. 13 – November 29, 2009
p. 63 – September 28, 2011
p. 66 – June 6, 2010
p. 67 – May 1, 2005
p. 71 – October 25, 2011
p. 74 – February 10, 2004
p. 75 – May 5, 2006
p. 98 – October 21, 2006
p. 99 – May 30, 2007
p. 101 – June 27, 2009
p. 101 – July 19, 2011
p. 139 – July 24, 2012
p. 145 – August 26, 2003
p. 147 – October 4, 2008
p. 155 – February 5, 2008
p. 168 – January 28, 2011
p. 171 – June 27, 2010

Bob Staake Illustrations: Published
originally at Bobstaake.com.
p. 137 – January 23, 2002

Strange Brew by John Deering:
Distributed to newspapers by Creators
Syndicate.
p. 142 – October 20, 2011

Ann Telnaes Editorial Cartoons:
Distributed to newspapers by
syndication.
p. xviii – July 25, 2004
p. 9 – September 30, 1997
p. 20 – November 25, 2006
p. 27 – January 19, 2000
p. 28 – April 17, 2008
p. 40 – February 1, 2004
p. 48 – October 29, 2003
p. 78 – January 4, 2002
p. 112 – December 7, 2004
p. 129 – December 27, 2003
p. 176 – April 27, 2008

That's Life by Mike Twohy:
Distributed to newspapers by the
Washington Post Writers Group.
p. 44 – February 16, 2004
p. 70 – March 3, 2003
p. 71 – December 23, 2004
p. 73 – January 18, 2007
p. 95 – February 18, 2003
p. 117 – December 6, 2006
p. 121 – December 4, 2006
p. 172 – August 16, 2004
p. 173 – August 23, 2004

Tina's Groove by Rina Piccolo:
Distributed to newspapers by King
Features Syndicate.
p. 61 – February 10, 2012

Gary Varvel Editorial Cartoons:
Published originally in the *Indianapolis
Star*.
p. 21 – October 26, 2011
p. 28 – May 2, 2008
p. 43 – May 26, 2010
p. 64 – February 17, 2011
p. 90 – November 20, 2011
p. 150 – April 22, 2010
p. 151 – May 14, 2009
p. 167 – July 18, 2012

**Signe Wilkinson Editorial
Cartoons:** Published originally in the
Philadelphia Daily News.
p. 22 – January 1, 1986
p. 23 – November 26, 2008
p. 24 – January 12, 2012
p. 46 – March 11, 2004
p. 54 – April 21, 2005
p. 57 – April 2, 2012
p. 78 – September 14, 2011
p. 81 – March 18, 2011
p. 81 – August 4, 2010
p. 85 – February 11, 2010
p. 100 – March 28, 2006
p. 128 – April 4, 2011
p. 132 – August 9, 2005
p. 154 – October 3, 2006
p. 157 – March 15, 2010
p. 159 – June 3, 2012

Matt Wuerker Editorial Cartoons:
Unless otherwise noted, distributed to
newspapers via syndication.
   p. 6 – May 21, 2008*
   *Published originally in Politico.
   p. 8 – April 2, 2004
   p. 10 – June 28, 2011*
   *Published originally in Politico.
   p. 25 – November 15, 2005
   p. 130 – January 7, 2004

**Zits by Jim Borgman and Jerry
Scott:** Distributed to newspapers by
King Features Syndicate.
   p. 61 – April 21, 2010

ADDITIONAL COPYRIGHTS

Nick Anderson Editorial Cartoons ©Nick
Anderson. Used with the permission of
Nick Anderson and the *Washington Post*
Writers Group in conjunction with The
Cartoonist Group. All rights reserved.

Arctic Circle ©Alex Hallatt. Used with
the permission of Alex Hallatt and
King Features Syndicate in conjunction
with The Cartoonist Group. All rights
reserved.

Baby Blues ©Baby Blues Partnership.
Used with the permission of the Baby
Blues Partnership and King Features
Syndicate in conjunction with The Car-
toonist Group. All rights reserved.

Clay Bennett Editorial Cartoons ©Clay
Bennett. Used with the permission of
Clay Bennett and the *Washington Post*
Writers Group in conjunction with The
Cartoonist Group. All rights reserved.

Lisa Benson Editorial Cartoons ©Lisa
Benson. Used with the permission of Lisa
Benson and the *Washington Post* Writers
Group in conjunction with The Cartoon-
ist Group. All rights reserved.

Bizarro ©Dan Piraro. Used with the permission of Dan Piraro and King Features
Syndicate in conjunction with The Cartoonist Group. All rights reserved.

Chip Bok Editorial Cartoons ©Chip
Bok. Used with the permission of Chip
Bok and Creators Syndicate. All rights
reserved.

Brilliant Mind of Edison Lee ©John
Hambrock. Used with the permission of
John Hambrock and King Features Syndicate in conjunction with The Cartoonist Group. All rights reserved.

Candorville ©Darrin Bell. Used with the
permission of Darrin Bell and the *Washington Post* Writers Group in conjunction
with The Cartoonist Group. All rights
reserved.

Jeff Danziger Editorial Cartoons ©Jeff
Danziger. Used with the permission of
Jeff Danziger and The Cartoonist Group.
All rights reserved.

John Deering Editorial Cartoons ©John
Deering. Used with the permission of
John Deering and Creators Syndicate. All
rights reserved.

Liza Donnelley Panel Cartoons ©Liza
Donnelley. Used with the permission
of Liza Donnelley and The Cartoonist
Group. All rights reserved.

Dustin ©Steve Kelley and Jeff Parker.
Used with the permission of Steve Kelley,
Jeff Parker, and King Features Syndi-
cate in conjunction with The Cartoonist
Group. All rights reserved.

Family Tree ©Signe Wilkinson. Used
with the permission of Signe Wilkinson
and The Cartoonist Group. All rights
reserved.

Frank and Ernest ©Thaves. Used with
the permission of the Thaves family
and The Cartoonist Group. All rights
reserved.

Lee Judge Editorial Cartoons ©Lee
Judge. Used with the permission of Lee
Judge and The Cartoonist Group. All
rights reserved.

Steve Kelley Editorial Cartoons ©Steve
Kelley. Used with the permission of Steve
Kelley and Creators Syndicate. All rights
reserved.

Luann ©GEC, Inc. Used with the permission of GEC, Inc. and The Cartoonist
Group. All rights reserved.

INDEX

Boldface page references indicate cartoons.

Also by Marion Nestle

Nutrition in Medical Practice (1985)

Food Politics: How the Food Industry Influences Nutrition and Health (2002; Tenth anniversary edition, with a foreword by Michael Pollan, 2013)

Safe Food: The Politics of Food Safety (2003, revised and expanded edition, 2010)

What to Eat (2006)

Pet Food Politics: The Chihuahua in the Coal Mine (2008)

Feed Your Pet Right (with Malden Nesheim) (2010)

Why Calories Count: From Science to Politics (with Malden Nesheim) (2012)

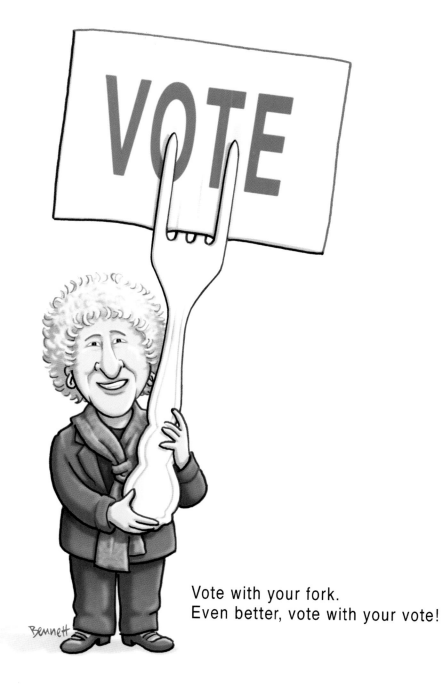

Vote with your fork.
Even better, vote with your vote!